First Edition 1997
ISBN 7-5331-1894-4

**Non-pharmacotherapies
for Diabetes**
Editor-in-Chief Cheng Yichun
Translators Zhang Yuxi
Lu Yubin
Editor-in-Charge Wang Weizhen
Zhong Pengjun

*

Published by Shandong Science and Technology Press
16 Yuhan Road, Jinan, China 250002
Distributed by China International Book Trading Corporation
35 Chegongzhuang Xilu, Beijing, China 100044
P. O. Box 399, Beijing, China
Printed in the Poeple's Republic of China

Non-pharmacotherapies for Diabetes

Editor-in-Chief Cheng Yichun
Translators Zhang Yuxi
Lu Yubin

SHANDONG SCIENCE AND TECHNOLOGY PRESS

Preface

Diabetes is a common and frequently-occurring disease whichendangers human health and lives. Unfortunately, its incidence tends torise year by year. It has been a troublesome problem to medicalscientists all over the world owing to its high lethality anddisability rate of the disease itself and its complications. Though manycountries put a considerable amount of funding into the study of thedisease every year, little effect has been produced. The complexity ofits etiology also renders it very difficult to prevent. In recent years, the study of the disease has developed into a new special discipline andmany scholars have devoted themselves to the deepening study of thedisease with regard to its etiology and pathology. Some new advanceshave been made both in traditional Chinese medicine (TCM) and inWestern medicine with a number of good methods for its prevention andtreatment. However, they are based, in most cases, on pharmacotherapyand physical exercise, and the unavailability of really effectivetherapeutic methods still embarrasses the medical world as well as thevictims of the disease.

Since most diabetics usually rely only on pharmacotherpay withoutdue attention to non-pharmacotherapies, their condition is often aggra-vated rapidly, which brings not only adverse impact on their physicaland mental health but also a great burden to their families and even thesociety. Therefore, we have compiled this book, concentrating on the introduction of non-pharmacotherapies such as psychotherapy, kinesitherapy, Qigong therapy, acupuncture and moxibustion therapy, etc. for theprevention and treatment of the disease with the hope that it can benefit both the clinical work and diabetics to make some contributions tohumanity.

Cheng Yichun
Deputy President of
the Affiliated Hospital to
Shandong College of TCM

Contents

General Situation of the Treatment of Diabetes 1
    Knowledge of Diabetes in Modern Medicine 2
    Knowledge of Diabetes in TCM 6
    Application of Non-pharmacotherapies for Diabetes 11

Psychotherapy in the Treatment of Diabetes 15
    A Brief Account of Psychotherapy 15
    The Theoretical Basis of TCM Psychotherapy 19
    The Causes of Psychological Disturbance in Diabetics 25
    The Characteristics of Psychological
    Disturbance of Diabetics 26
    Common Psychotherapy Methods
    in the Treatment of Diabetes 30
    Attaching Importance to Psychological
    Care for Diabetics 37

Dietotherapy for Diabetes 40
    The Concept of Dietotherapy 40
    The Aim of Dietotherapy 41
    The Basic Principles of Dietotherapy 42
    The Control of Total Calorie Intake 44
    The Dietary Calculation and Diet Planning 47
    Points for Attention in Dietotherapy 51
    Foods Often Used to Treat Diabetes 55
    Simple Food Recipes Commonly Used for Diabetes 59

Kinesitherapy for Diabetes 65
  A Brief Introduction of
  Kinesitherapy for Diabetes 65
  The Beneficial Effects of Physical
  Exercise on Diabetics 66
  Adverse Effects of Improper Physical
  Exercise on Diabetics 69
  The Indications of Kinesitherapy 70
  Contraindications to Kinesitherapy 71
  Points for Attention During Kinesitherapy 71
  Contents and Methods of Kinesitherapy 72

Qigong Therapy for Diabetes 77
  A Brief Account of Qigong Therapy 77
  Mechanism of Qigong Therapy 86
  Present Situation and Advances of Qigong Therapy
  in the Treatment of Diabetes 95
  Contents and Methods of Qigong Therapy
  in the Treatment of Diabetes 98
  Points for Attention in Qigong Therapy 113

Acupuncture and Moxibustion Treatment For Diabetes 119
  A Brief Account About Acupuncture and Moxibustion
  in the Treatment of Diabetes 119
  Mechanism of Acupuncture and Moxibustion
  in the treatment of Diabetes 122
  Present Situation of Research on Acupuncture and
  Moxibustion in the treatment of Diabetes 127
  Methods of Acupuncture and Moxibustion
  in the Treatment of Diabetes 134

Points of Attention In the Treatment of Diabetes
with Acupuncture and Moxibustion 155

Massotherapy In the Treatment of Diabetes 156
   A Brief Account of Massotherapy 156
   Mechanism of Massotherapy 158
   Clinical Application of Massotherapy 160
   Points of Attention in the Treatment
   of Diabetes with Massotherapy 166

General Situation of the Treatment of Diabetes

Diabetes is a common endocrine metabolic disease, which, due to its high incidence and numerous complications, is seriously detrimental to people's health. Now in some developed countries, diabetes has already ranked as the third on the list of the major diseases, next only to tumors and cardiocerebrovascular diseases. According to statistics, there are now about 120 million diabetic patients in the world, and it is estimated that this figure will rise year by year with the development of economy, advances of society, improvement of living standard along with the aggravation of such socio-environmental factors as intense work, overstress, and hyperalimentation. For many years, thousands and thousands of medical scientists all over the world have devoted themselves to the study of the disease. Although there has been no big breakthrough since the discovery of insulin in 1921, great advances have been made in this study. Artificial islets of pancreas, pancreatic islets transplantation and the invention of a new generation of numerous hypoglycemic agents have remarkably enhanced the therapeutic effects of the treatment of diabetes. However, due to the lack of clarity of the causes and pathogenesis of the disease, its treatment still lingers at the level of expectant treatment focussing on lowering glucose level in blood and urine. There is not yet any effective causal treatment, nor effective preventive measures for its complications. Therefore, most scientists believe that at present it is preferable to treat diabetes with a comprehensive treatment, that is, in addition to pharmacotherapy, such remedies as dietotherapy, kinesitherapy, physicotherapy, acupuncture and moxibustion and massotherapy should be administered. The comprehensive treatment not only intensifies the therapeutic effect for diabetes but also prevents various complications.

Knowledge of Diabetes in Modern Medicine

1. What is diabetes

Diabetes is a generalized disorder of endocrine metabolism due to an absolute or relative deficiency of insulin secretion, characterized clinically by excessive thirst, an increase in appetite, excessive urine, emaciation and abnormal excess of glucose in the blood, and pathologically by disturbance of carbohydrate metabolism at the early stage and subsequent disturbance of fat and protein metabolism. As the disease develops, it may result in chronic progressive pathologic change in the tissues of many vital organs such as the heart, blood vessels of the brain, kidneys, eyes, nerves, etc. If the disease goes without proper and prompt treatment, blindness, gangrene of the lower limbs, uremia, cerebrovascular accident and heart lesion tend to occur, which are the main causes of death or disability. Emergent and serious complications like diabetic ketoacidosis, hyperosmotic nonketonic coma, and lactic acidosis may develop in a few diabetics to endanger their lives.

2. Types of diabetes

Diabetes is classified by the World Health Organization (WHO) into the following types:

(1) Insulin-dependent diabetes mellitus (also referred to as IDDM, Type I): Diabetics of this type account for 5%-10% of the total diabetic patients, most of them being young children and juveniles. This kind of diabetes is characterized by a sudden onset with marked symptoms of excessive thirst, abnormal increase of

appetite, excessive urine and general weakness. The plasma insulin level in such patients is lower than normal so the patient has to depend on exogenetic insulin treatment, the suspension of which is apt to lead to diabetic ketoacidosis and aggravate the disease.

(2) Non-insulin-dependent diabetes mellitus (also referred to as NIDDM, Type II): Diabetics of this type account for about 80%-90% of the total diabetic patients. In most cases, the disorder occurs to individuals over 40 years old. The onset is usually chronic and the condition mild. The symptoms of excessive thirst, abnormal increase of appetite, excessive urine, and general weakness are usually not remarkable. With the endogenous insulin level being normal, or slightly below or above normal, patients are not dependent on exogenetic insulin treatment and the administration of a hypoglycemic agent will usually do. Insulin treatment is necessary only when the condition is severe.

In addition to the above mentioned types, there are secondary diabetes and dystrophic diabetes. The former follows other diseases or results from over-administration of certain drugs. The latter is rare, and is reported time and again in the developing countries in the tropical zone.

3. Causes and pathogenesis

The causes of the disease still remain unclear. It may have some relationship with the following factors: intrinsic factors, including hereditary background, race, constitution, immunity, and individual neuroendocrine regulation, and extrinsic factors involving diet habit, nutrition, obesity, mental stress, viral infection and chemicals. The interaction between the intrinsic and extrinsic factors may cause the disorder. Most researchers now assume that IDDM occurs when initiating pathogenic factors (e.g. viral infection), on the basis of hereditary susceptibility, damage the islet β-cells first to cause denaturation of the β-cell protein, which, as a sensitizing protein, then triggers a generalized immunological reaction. This reaction further damages the islet β-cells to cause an absolute deficiency of insulin secretion, which will in turn result in hyperglycemia to cause IDDM. In the case of NIDDM, it is also under the joint actions of such factors as genetic diathesis, obesity and mental stress that defect of islet β-cells, defect of insulin receptors, post-receptor defect and increase of insulin antagonistic hormones develop, which go on to give rise to pathological changes such as retardation of insulin secretion, insulin resistance, and increase in the output of hepatic glucose so that relative deficiency of insulin secretion occurs to cause NIDDM.

4. Diagnosis

At present, the diagnostic criteria for diabetes drawn up by WHO in 1980 are popularly adopted in the world (i.e. determination of plasma glucose with glucose-oxidase).

(1) Symptomatic diabetes: ① The concentration of fasting blood-glucose$\geqslant$7.8mmol/L, or at any time of the day, the blood-glucose value $\geqslant$11.1mmol/L; ② Fasting blood-glucose value $<$ 7.8mmol/L but in glucose tolerance test, blood-glucose value in two hours$\geqslant$ 11.1 mmol/L. The diagnosis can be established when either of the two criteria is positive.

(2) Asymptomatic diabetes: ① Fasting blood-glucose value$\geqslant$ 7.8mmol/L in two tests; ② In glucose tolerance test, blood-glucose value in two hours$\geqslant$11.1mmol/L; in a repetition of the glucose tolerance test, blood-glucose value in two hours$\geqslant$11.1mmol/L or in a repetition of fasting blood-glucose test, blood-glucose value$\geqslant$7.8mmol/L. The diagnosis can be made when either of the tests is positive.

(3) Decrease of glucose tolerance: When fasting blood-glucose $\leqslant$7.8mmol/L, and in the glucose tolerance test, blood-glucose within two hours is 7.8-11.1.mmol/L, the diagnosis can be established.

5. Treatment

Since in any type of diabetes, the insulin provided by islets can not meet the demands of the target tissues in the metabolism of glucose, fats and proteins, the treatment, therefore, aims at restoring the balance between supply and demand of insulin so as to maintain the normal metabolism and prevent development of complications. In modern medicine, the treatment of diabetes consists of mainly three therapies: diet control (dietotherapy), moderate physical exercise (kinesitherapy) and medication (pharmacotherapy). Dietotherapy and kinesitherapy will be discussed fully in later chapters. Pharmacotherapy is chiefly composed of oral administration of hypoglycemic agents and insulin treatment. There are two major classes of oral hypoglycemic drugs: sulfaurea and biguanide drugs. The principal actions of the sulfaureas are stimulating the islet β-cells to secrete intrinsic insulin, limiting the output of hepatic glycogen and promoting the functions of insulin receptors in peripheral tissues. They are used in the treatment of NIDDM that is not satisfactorily controlled only with dietotherapy and kinesitherapy. Tolbutamide (D_{860}), Glybenzcyclamide (Euglucan), Diamicron, Glibornuride, Glipizide and Gliquidone are the common drugs of this group. The biguanides, such as Phenethyldiguanide and Dimethyldiguanide, take effects mainly by inhibiting the intestinal absorption of glucose and output of hepatic glycogen and by promoting the utilization of glucose in the peripheral tissues. Their indications include: ① NIDDM of obesity type; ② IDDM with unsatisfactory response to insulin treatment; ③ Secondary ineffectiveness of sulfaureas, in which case biguanide drugs are used as a supplement. Insulin preparations are classified into short-acting, medium-term-acting and long-acting. Their indications include: ① IDDM; ② NIDDM not under satisfactory control after dietotherapy and oral administration of hypoglycemic agents; ③ Diabetes complicated by ketoacidosis, hyperosmotic nonketonic coma, lactic acidosis, severe infection and progressive retinopathy, and diabetic renopathy, acute myocardial infarction, and cerebrovascular accident; ④ Diabetic patients before or after an operation, or during pregnancy and at the stages of labor.

However, although medicaments are effective in treating diabetes, they also have the disadvantages of secondary ineffectiveness and various side effects. Moreover, more effective drugs for the chronic complications of diabetes are still to be found.

Knowledge of Diabetes in TCM

The study of diabetes in TCM has a long histroty. In *The Yellow Emperor's Internal Classic* written more than 2 000 years ago, there are records about the disease and a brief description about its causes and pathogenesis. In *The Golden Chamber of Medicine* by the famous ancient doctor Zhang Zongjing, a special chapter was devoted to the study of the disease. Wang Tao, a famous physician in the Tang Dynasty, quoted in his medical book *The Medical Secrets from an Official* from an earlier medical book *Proved Recipes from the Ancient Times* the following: "If one who feels excessively thirsty, drinks a lot of water and passes urine very frequently which resembles wheat bran and tastes sweet, he is undoubtedly suffering from diabetes." Here the special feature of diabetes—the urine is sweet—is pointed out. This discovery is more than 1 000 years earlier than that made by Western medicine. In the Song, Ming and Qing dynasties, most physicians set much store on the treatment of diabetes by further dividing it into diabetes involving the upper Jiao, diabetes involving the middle Jiao and diabetes involving the lower Jiao and laid special emphasis on the regulation of kidney functions. In short, every generation of physicians of TCM have given accounts of the causes, pathogenesis and treatment, of the disorder, and much of their understanding and many of their views are still of guiding significance in the treatment of the disease. By mastering the quintessence from ancient literature and combining it with their knowledge of modern medicine, and on the basis of basic experiments, modern medical scientists have laboured at further studies and treatment of diabetes and have achieved great advances, which are presented as follows:

1. **Causes and pathogenesis**

The medical theories in ancient TCM literature and modern studies in Chinese medicine show little differences on the causes of the disease, which are held to be connected with the following factors: weak constitution, unrestrained diet, emotional imbalances, overstrain, hypererosia, and toxicity of drugs taken and alcoholic drinks. However, there are differences on the understanding of pathogenesis. The following are the main viewpoints:

(1) Diabetes results from Yin deficiency and internal dryness-heat: This is the traditional view of TCM in treating diabetes, and has constantly been an important guiding principle in clinical diagnosis and treatment. It is generally believed that many pathogenic factors first result in excessive dryness-heat in the body and consumption of body fluids, which in turn work on each other as the mutual causation to give rise to diabetes. The disorder has much to do with the lungs, spleen, stomach and mainly with the kidneys. Chronic diabetes may lead to impairment to both Qi and Yin and a deficiency of both Yin and Yang.

(2) Diabetes is due to a deficiency of both Qi and Yin: Many physicians believe that the pathologic change of this disease is mainly caused by a deficiency of both Qi and Yin. Pathogenic factors may render the internal organs deficient in Qi, which can cause disturbance in the formation, transformation, distribution and excretion, of Yin fluids (including various kinds of body fluids such as blood, saliva and spermatic fluid) and food essence. As a result, the Yin fluids and food essence cannot circulate all over the body through their normal systems but are excreted in great quantity with the urine. If the condition lasts long, Qi will become more deficient. As a result, Qi and Yin are unable to hold each other together and maintain availability of their mutual support. This is where the crux lies that diabetes is difficult to cure.

(3) Diabetes is due to accumulation of blood stasis: The relationship between diabetes and blood stasis was already explained in ancient literature such as *The Yellow Emperor's Internal Classic*, and *The Golden Chamber of Medicine*. In recent years, many researchers have found in their studies that in most cases of diabetes, signs of blood stasis can be noticed on examination of the tongue picture, and that high tendency of blood coagulation, greater blood viscosity and microcirculatory disturbance are pre-

sent. These pathologic changes conincide with the pathogenesis described by the TCM that "inadequate circulatory mobility will lead to accumulation of blood stasis." The pathogenic machanism may be due to a deficiency of Qi so that Qi is unable to command the blood, due to a deficiency of Yin so that there is consumption of body fluids and due to the scorching by the excessive internal heat.

(4) Diabetes is due to a spleen deficiency: The spleen has the function to transform and transport nutrients. It helps digest food, absorb food essence and distribute the nutrients to tissues and structures all over the body and nourish them. So the deficiency of the spleen can be assumed as the pathogenesis of diabetes. When the Spleen Qi is deficient, the spleen loses the functions of transforming and transporting nutrients and fails to distribute nutrients to the whole body, and instead, lets them go down to the bladder and be discharged with urine. The result is diabetes marked by the typical three "poly-" symptoms (polydipsia, polyphagia and polyuria) and one "lack" symptom (lack of strength).

(5) Diabetes is due to the stagnation of Liver Qi: The liver has the function of smoothing and regulating the flow and operation of Qi. Emotional disturbance or fury can affect the functioning of the liver, which may also lead to functional disturbances of the lung, spleen, stomach and other viscera. It is found statistically that most diabetics, prior to their disease, have undergone such emotional irritation as mental stress and depression.

2. Treatments on the basis of differentiation of syndromes

The traditional treatment of the disease in TCM is usually carried out by distinguishing which of the three "poly's" is the primary symptom and which is the secondary to sort the disease into three types and to treat it accordingly. Diabetes involving the upper Jiao marked primarily by polydipsia is treated with *Baihu Tang* (White Tiger Decoction) plus *Rensheng Tang* (Decoction of Ginseng) or modified *Xiaoke Fang* (Decoction for Diabetes). Diabetes involving the middle Jiao, marked chiefly by polyphagia and constant hunger, is attributed to excess heat in the stomach and is treated with *Yunu Jian* (Gypsum Decoction) or modified *Sanhuang Tang* (Decoction of Radix Coptidis, Radix Scutellariae and Cortex Phellodendri). Diabetes involving the lower Jiao marked mainly by polyuria and attributed to deficiency of kidney is treated with *Liuwei Dihuang Wan* (Bolus of Six Drugs Including Rehmannia) or modified *Jingui Shenqi Wan* (Pills for Restoring Vital Energy and Functions of the Kidney). However, the above traditional three-type division and management cannot satisfy the clinical needs because the pathogenesis of the disease is often so complicated, the pathological changes often involve so many aspects like Yin, Yang, Qi, blood and more than one visceral organ, and the patient's constitution, the course and the condition of the disease vary so much that clinically the disease is usually of a complicated nature: symptoms and signs of both deficiency and excess types, imbalance between Yin and Yang, disharmony of Qi and blood, and symptoms of the three types of diabetes may all be present at the same time. In recent years, therefore, many doctors have tried to classify and treat the disease on the basis of differentiation between Yin and Yang, Qi and blood, and between the visceral organs. The classification reveals the pathogenesis more accurately and is, therefore, beneficial to clinical treatment. At present, diabetes is classified into the following four types for treatment:

(1) Diabetes due to Yin deficiency and dryness-heat: This type of diabetes is characterized by excessive thirst, polyphagia with a tendency to hunger, feverish feeling in the palms and soles, constipation, red tongue with little fur, lack of saliva, thready and rapid pulse. The therapeutic strategy for this type is nourishing Yin and removing heat. *Yuquan San* (Jade Spring Powder) or modified *Baihu Tang* (White Tiger Decoction) enforced by *Renshen Tang* (Ginseng Decoction) is often prescribed for the treatment.

(2) Diabetes due to deficiency of both Qi and Yin: It is marked by dry mouth and throat, polydipsia, polyuria, emaciation, lack

of strength, being short of breath, spontaneous sweating, red tongue with little fur and rapid thready and weak pulse. The principle of treatment is supplementing Qi and nourishing Yin. *Shengmai San* (Pulse-activating Powder) in combination with *Liuwei Dihuang Wan* (Bolus of Six Drugs Including Rehmmania) or modified *Yuye Tang* (Decoction for Promoting Secretion of Saliva) should be prescribed.

(3) Diabetes due to accumulation of blood stasis: It is manifested as dry mouth and thirst, emaciation, lack of strength, or chest distress and pain, numbness and pain in the limbs, dizziness, headache, blurred vision, darkened tongue with petechiae or ecchymosis and thready and unsmooth pulse. The treatment focuses on invigorating blood circulation to remove blood stasis. The prescriptions commonly used are *Shengmai San* (Pulse-activating Powder) in combination with *Buyang Huanwu Tang* (Decoction Invigorating Yang for Recuperation), and modified *Taohe Chengqi Tang* (Decoction of Peach Kernel for Activating Qi).

(4) Diabetes due to deficiency of both Yin and Yang: This type is characterized by frequent nocturia, dizziness, tinnitus, lassitude in the loin and legs, impotence, diarrhea, aversion to cold, cold limbs, pale tongue with white coating, and deep thready weak pulse. It is treated by tonifying kidney and warming Yang, and modified *Jingui Shenqi Wan* (Pills for Restoring Vital Energy and Functions of the Kidney) is usually prescribed for the patient.

The types mentioned above and their corresponding treatments are just the ways commonly used in clinical practice at present. However, when it comes to any individual, the treatment should vary on the basis of differentiation of his symptoms and signs, his constitution, the causes, etc. Only in such a way can satisfactory therapeutic effect be achieved.

3. Simple recipes and proved recipes

Many simple and proved recipes are of desirable effect on the disease. It has been proved that the following individual drugs exhibit remarkable hypoglycemic effect: *Radix Ginseng*, *Radix Astragali seu Hedysary*, *Rhizoma Coptidis*, *Radix Rehmanni-*

ae, *Cortex Lycii Radicis*, *Semen Litchi*, *Bombyx Batriticatus*, *Fructus Lycii*, *Rhizoma Polygonati*, *Rhizoma Dioscoreae*, *Stigma Maydis*, *Concha Ostreae*, *Fructus Psidii Guajavae Immaturus*, *Fructus Momordicae Charantiae*, *Fructus Cucurbitae*, etc.

There are also many compound prescriptions for the treatment of this disease, such as *Xiaokeping Pian* (Tablet for Diabetes), *Jiawei Taohe Chengqi Tang* (Modified Decoction of Peach Kernel for Activating Qi), *Zishen Rongjing Wan* (Pill for Replenishing the Kidney Yin and Vitality), *Jiangtang Wan* (Hypoglycemic Pill), *Xiaoke Wan* (Pill for Diabetes), etc. They have proved in experiments and clinical observations to possess nice therapeutic effects for both diabetes and its complications.

Application of Non-pharmacotherapies for Diabetes

Since diabetes is a syndrome of metabolic disturbance of glucose, fat and protein, it involves many systems and viscera and has a close relationship with such factors as social environment, psychology, diet habits and sports. Many medical scientists, therefore, suggest that a comprehensive treatment of non-pharmacotherapies, including dietotherapy, psycotherapy, kinesitherapy, acupuncture and moxibustion therapy and massotherapy, as well as pharmacotherapy, be adopted so that desirable therapeutic effects can be achieved. It has been found that all drugs which are widely used at present for treating diabetes have some toxic or side effects which may sometimes result in certain drug-induced diseases. Therefore, man is searching for a treatment that will not produce toxic or side effects. Especially in the strong cry that "man should return to nature", non-pharmacotherapies without adverse effects are becoming favoured by more and more people.

In fact non-pharmacotherapies have a very long history. Early in the remote antiquity man began to use stone needles and bone needles to treat diseases. In the earliest medical work extant in China, *The Yellow Emperor's Internal Classic*, which was written in the Warring States Period (475-221 BC), non-pharmacotherapies were recorded, such as acupuncture and moxibustion, dietotherapy, psychotherapy, massotherapy, and *Daoyin* (a physical and breathing exercise), whose indications and methods were also described therein. And what is more, the basic theories like viscera-state doctrine, the meridian doctrine, Qi and blood theory, etc. established in *The Yellow Emperor's Internal Classic* laid the theoretical foundation for the development of non-pharmacotherapies. Medical scientists of all generations thereafter have extensively applied, on the basis of *The Yellow Emperor's Internal Classic*, non-pharmacotherapies to treat diseases, and greatly developed and improved them so that they are becoming better and approaching perfection day by day in the basic theories and clinical practice. For example, large amounts of records about non-pharmacotherapies can be found in later books, like *Shen Nong's Herbal Classic*, *Treatise on Febrile and Miscellaneous Diseases*, *A-B Classic of Acupuncture and Moxibustion*, *Essential Prescriptions Worth a Thousand Gold*, *A Dietetic Materia Medica*, and *Compendium of Materia Medica*. In recent decades, in the popularization of non-pharmacotherapies, great successes have been scored in their systematization, research and clinical practice, especially in dietotherapy, acupuncture and moxibustion, and massage. Now non-pharmacotherapies are becoming more and more important in clinical practice.

Ancient people also applied non-pharmacotherapies in the treatment of diabetes. Sun Simiao, a renowned physician and Taoist (581-682 AD) of the Tang Dynasty stated in the chapter "Diabetes" in his book *Essential Prescriptions Worth a Thousand Gold*: "Whether a diabetic patient can be cured or not depends on whether he is prudent in the following things: drinking, sex and salty and flour food. If he is prudent enough about them, he will be alright even though he does not take any medicine; otherwise, the best medicine cannot cure him of his illness. Therefore, one must think deeply about the truth and be prudent in practice." Another renowned ancient physician, Zhang Zihe, also mentioned in his book *Confucians' Duties to their Parents*: "If a diabetic, after recovery, does not limit his desires for food, give up his addictions and refrain himself from excessive joy and anger, his disease is bound to have a relapse. On the contrary, if he is able to fulfill these three things, he needn't worry about his diabetes." He explicitly stated the importance of control of diet, emotions, sex and addictions in the treatment of diabetes. The famous physician Chao Yuanfang of the Sui Dynasty (550-630 AD) already knew that moderate physical exercise is an important method in the treatment of diabetes. In his work *General Treatise on the Etiology and Symptoms of Diseases*, he advocated: "A diabetic should walk at least 120 steps, or as many as one thousand steps prior to a meal." Wang Tao wrote in his work *Medical Secrets from an Official* that diabetics should "have a walk after a meal and not sit until the abdomen is comfortable."

Acupuncture and moxibustion, one of the gems of traditional Chinese medicine, has long been playing an important role in the treatment of diabetes. Huangfu Mi of the Jin Dynasty wrote in his book *A-B Classic of Acupuncture and Moxibustion*: "For diabetes marked by fever and reddish yellow complexion, puncture the acupoint Yishe. If it is marked by polydipsia, puncture Chengjiang; if marked by sleepiness and lassitude of the limbs, puncture Wangu; if marked by a deficiency of Yin, heat in the middle Jiao, and polyorexia, puncture Zusanli." In *Essential Prescriptions Worth a Thousand Gold*, *Medical Secrets from an Official* and other ancient medical books, there are detailed descriptions about the treatment of diabetes with acupuncture and moxibustion.

In short, medical scientists of past generations have made a great deal of exposition on the treatment of diabetes with therapies other than medication and by constant development, enrichment and perfection of all the therapies in clinical practice, and have formulated a system of effective treatments.

It is believed in TCM that dietotherapy, psychotherapy, Qigong, acupuncture and moxibustion, massage and other non-pharmacotherapies are theoretically based on TCM's wholism concept of correspondence between man and the universe, viscera theory, meridian doctrine, Yin-Yang theory, Qi and blood theory and autoploidy of medicine and food. These non-pharmacotherapies are effective in strengthening body resistance and eliminating pathogenic factors, regulating the balance between Yin and Yang, reinforcing the viscera and reducing pathogenic factors, regulating the function of Qi, dredging the channels and collaterals, etc., so that the aim of eliminating diseases and prolonging life span can be achieved. The non-pharmacotherapy concept is also identical with the new nature-man-society mode of medicine. Research work of modern medicine has already proved that non-pharmacotherapies produce good two-way regulatory effects on all the major body systems, and thus increase the body's immunity, promote the metabolism of glucose, fat and protein, improve blood circulation and regulate the functions of the whole body. They exhibit more remarkable effects particularly in the treatment of psychophysical diseases like diabetes and cerebrovascular diseases. Since they cure diseases chiefly by exciting the body's own natural vitality and regulating the body's internal balance, they have no side effects, and integrate prevention, treatment, rehabilitation, health care into one. As already mentioned before, non-pharmacotherapies are characterized by their wide indications, simplicity, convenience and easiness for use, economy and effectiveness, so they are popularly received. Along with the evergrowing popularization of dietotherapy, acupuncture and moxibustion, Qigong, and massage on the worldwide scale, there will be a considerable increase all over the world in the medical respectability of the treatment of diabetes with non-pharmacotherapies, which will make a great contribution to an early understanding and successful treatment of this difficult and complicated disease—diabetes.

Psychotherapy in the Treatment of Diabetes

A Brief Account of Psychotherapy

1. The implications of psychotherapy

Psychotherapy here refers to a therapeutic regime adopted, in the course of his treatment of a patient, by a doctor who uses his psychological knowledge to help his patient alleviate or even get rid of his illness. It belongs to the category of non-pharmacotherapies.

Owing to the varying understanding of the connotation and denotation of the concept of psychotherapy, it is generally thought to have a narrow sense, an intermediate sense and a broad sense.

Psychotherapy in a narrow sense refers to a treatment which, with "words" as the basic means, takes advantage of the therapeutic effects of speech to relieve a patient of his symptoms and pain. Its typical way of treatment is verbal enlightening.

Psychotherapy in the intermediate sense refers to a way of treatment that, in the course of conversation with his patient, the doctor, with his words, attitude and behavior, influences and changes the patient's feeling, understanding, mood, attitude and behavior to relieve or eliminate the emotions and behaviors which have caused the patient's mental agony and physical symptoms. This is a kind of psychotherapy parallel to surgical treatment, medical treatment, acupuncture and moxibustion treatment, physiotherapy, etc. It includes many kinds of treatment like verbal enlightening, analytic psychotherapy, behavior therapy, and work and recreational therapy. Unlike acupuncture, moxibustion, medicine and surgery, which act directly on the body in visible forms, psychotherapy acts on the patient's psychology through sense organs in an invisible form to produce therapeutic effects.

Psychotherapy in the broad sense refers to a method which gives positive influence on the patient's psychology by various means and through all kinds of ways. It covers the following aspects: Firstly, every doctor, no matter whether he is a psychiatrist, a physician, a surgeon, a gynecologist or a pediatrician, will conduct psychotherapy consciously or unconsciously in the course of contact and conversation with the patient and during examination. Secondly, in the course of treatment, psychotherapy will be given as the principal means but such auxilliary treatment as acupuncture and medicine are not excluded. Lastly, under the guidance but without actual participation of the doctor, the patient himself consciously makes active psychological adjustment to cure his disease.

The psychotherapy discussed in this book refers to psychotherapy in the broad sense. It includes the contents of psychotherapy in the narrow sense and in the intermediate sense. In the therapy, both the doctor and patient play their parts, which is true of the TCM's dialectical and unified concept of wholism.

2. The features of TCM psychotherapy

Psychotherapy is the science dealing with the occurrence, development and changes of human psychological activities. The TCM Psychology is the science which, in the light of TCM theories and by application of the basic knowledge of psychology, deals with what roles psychologic factors play in the occurrence and development of diseases in the human body and the law in the course of diagnosis, treatment and prevention. It is a new branch of science evolved from the combination of TCM and psychology. TCM Psychotherapy is the therapeutic method which makes use of

TCM theories and psychological knowledge to prevent and treat human diseases so as to relieve patients of their diseases and pain. Since TCM is an independent system, the psychotherapy of TCM exhibits the following innate features:

(1) Oriental dialectical ideology: As is known, TCM has developed in the background of ancient oriental culture and science. Its viscera state doctrine, meridian doctrine, the concepts of Jing (essence of life), Qi (vital energy) and Shen (vitality), and other concepts are formulated on the basis of the theories of Yin-Yang and five evolusive elements. It is, therefore, no wonder that the contents of TCM psychotherapy bear a strong color of oriental culture. And just because of this oriental scientific background, TCM psychotherapy has its distinctive characteristics. For instance, the mode of thinking and way of practice manifested by the understanding of dialectical unity of the antagonistic and interdependent relations of Yin and Yang and their mutual transformation, and the promoting, checking, encroching and violating relations between the five evolusive elements, are up to the present still advanced in some aspects. The emotion-overcome-emotion treatment in TCM psychotherapy is theoretically based on the dialectical ideology of the concept of five evolusive elements.

(2) Individual difference: One of the clinical characteristics of TCM is making a diagnosis and prescribing treatment on the basis of an overall analysis of symptoms and signs, the cause, nature and location of the illness and the patient's physical condition according to the basic theories of TCM. That is, attention should be paid to the influence by weather or climate, and geographic environment, and much importance should be attached to the patient's mental and physical variation and his reactive state, and different treatment should be given according to a patient's different condition. Since psychotherapy stresses individual differences, the proposition that individual differences should be emphasized in the course of diagnosis and treatment based on the overall analysis of the patient's condition in TCM is very beneficial to the development of psychotherapy. The theory of Yin and Yang types of per-

sonality and constitution in TCM, for example, is the best embodiment of this viewpoint of individual differences. According to the different characteristics of a patient's disease caused by emotional disturbance and an overall analysis of his actual condition, different methods of psychotherapy can be adopted, such as bipolarity repeating method, opposite emotion method and emotion-overcome-emotion method.

(3) The wholism concept in treatment: The concept of wholism is another charateristic of TCM. Since everyone has emotions and thoughts, a doctor is required to treat him dynamically and analyse his symptoms and signs, make the diagnosis, work out the therapeutic plan and perform treatment with a comprehensive point of view. This concept is reflected in the practice of psychotherapy as emphasis on the regulation and treatment of the whole body. From a point of view that the body and spirit are an organic entity in the practice of psychotherapy, it is required that attention should be paid to the reaction of spirit on the physical body. For example, it is by dealing with the "spirit" that the TCM psychotherapy methods, such as passion release therapy, therapy of relieving psychogenic factor, desirability fancy therapy, and therapy of grafting spirit to alter Qi, cure patients of their physical diseases. Furthermore, the wholism concept in treatment is also manifested in the application of the comprehensive treatment with psychotherapy as the chief means and medicaments, acupuncture and moxibustion as the adjuvant.

3. The necessity and importance of psychotherapy in the treatment of diabetes

In the past, the study of diabetes followed the train of thought of biomedicine pattern, and was conducted from the angles of molecular biology and pathologic anatomy so that diabetes was believed to be due to absolute or relative insufficiency of insulin secretion caused by viral infection, disturbance of genetic genes, hypoimmunity, and insulin resistance. So etiologically, the important actions of social, environmental and psychological factors on diabetics were neglected. As a result, its treatment was conducted purely from the angle of biomedicine, with oral administration of hypoglycemic agents or injection of insulin as the chief means of treatment, the therapeutic effects of which are neither stable nor desirable.

In recent years, the introduction of biology-psychology-sociology medicine pattern has brought about a new mode of thinking about the study of diabetes. It has been found through research that the etiology of diabetes has something to do not only with the physio-pathological factors but also with social, environmental and psychological factors. For instance, long-term overstress in work or study, disharmony in interpersonal relationships, pessimal stimulation by misfortunes in life, are all significant factors for the development and aggravation of diabetes. It has further been found upon clinical observations that most diabetics have, apart from the symptoms and manifestations of polydipsia, polyphagia, polyuria, emaciation and hyperglycemia, varying degrees of psychological disturbances and emotional abnormality, such as excessive worry, vexation, restlessness, nervousness, easy fright, impatience, irritability, sadness and liability to tears. For such patients, pure pharmacotherapy like oral administration of hypoglycemic agents or injection of insulin often fails to bring about an ideal result, but if psychotherapy is given at the same time, desirable effects that pharmacotherapy alone is unable to achieve are often ensured. In the treatment of diabetes, importance must be attached to the elimination of the pessimal socio-environmental stimulations to restore the abnormal psychological state to normal. With this as the prerequisite, medicaments may be given to treat the patient both psychologically and physically and satisfactory results can be achieved. For these reasons psychotherapy is of great importance in the treatment of diabetes

The Theoretical Basis of TCM Psychotherapy

How do the psychological activities occur and which organ does this function belong to? What is the relationship between psychological activities and physiological activities? What is the relationship between psychological activities and pathological changes? For these questions, TCM has a whole set of unique theories which provide the theoretical basis for TCM psychotherapy.

1. The seven emotion theory

It is believed in TCM that the seven emotions, i.e. joy, anger, melancholy, anxiety, grief, fear and terror, are the external reflection of the psychological response of a man to environmental stimuli. If an emotion is too violent, it may become a pathogenic factor. It is stated in the chapter "Grand Discussion on the Concept of Yin and Yang" in the book *Plain Questions*: "In the human body there are five viscera which produce five emotions: joy, anger, grief, melancholy and fear. Joy and anger may cause impairment to Qi, cold and heat cause damage to the physical figure, fury causes damages to Yin, and overjoy hurts Yang. If overjoy and fury are not properly restrained, it is difficult for one to keep a healthy life."

To overcome one emotion with another is an important means used in the treatment of diseases. It is believed in TCM that the law of promoting, checking, encroaching and violating of the five evolusive elements can be employed as an important means of psychotherapy for some diseases. Again as stated in the chapter "Grand Discussion on the Concept of Yin and Yang", "Anger causes impairment to the liver, but grief can overcome it"; "joy causes impairment to the heart and fear can overcome it"; "anxiety impairs the spleen, but anger can overcome it"; "melancholy impairs the lung but joy can overcome it" and "fear impairs the kidney but anxiety can overcome it." The psychotherapy of overcoming one emotion with another is based theoretically on the seven emotion theory and the law of interrelationships of the five evolusive elements in TCM.

2. The temperament-type theory

Diseases are caused by the action of long and violent stimulation from the external environment on the human body. However, the same stimulation to different individuals may cause diseases easily in some but not in others. And as far as those affected are concerned, the same stimulation to them may cause different types of diseases, and the diseases provoked may be of varying degrees and of different natures—cold, heat, deficiency or excess, which can be ascribed to the different types of temperament of individuals. When people of different types of temperament are subjected to a same pathogenic stimulus, their diseases will be of different types, nature, severity and manifestations of psychological disturbances. The psychotherapy of TCM is based on this temperament theory. Different types of temperament may be attributed chiefly to different congenital endowments. Generally speaking, people who are born insufficient and weak are susceptible to illnesses.

As to the study of types of human temperament, there are descriptions in *The Yellow Emperor's Internal Classic*, the earliest medical classic extant in China. In "On Natural Endowment" and "Twenty-five Kinds of People According to Yin and Yang", two chapters in *Miraculous Pivot*, there are not only systematic descriptions of the types of temperament and psychological features of people of different temperament, but also detailed analysis of different kinds of diseases people of different temperaments tend to suffer, and full descriptions of the treatment of these diseases. These records are highly valued by the medical and psychological professions.

3. The theory of unity of body and spirit

"Body" here refers to the physical configuration, including human physical body, constitution, i. e. the physiological functions. "Spirit" here refers to the mind, consciousness and expression, including senses, memory, thinking, feelings, will and other psychological activities. In TCM, body (represented by physiological activities) and spirit (represented by psychological activities) have long been associated as a whole, that is to say, the body and spirit are interdependent, interacting, closely interrelated and inseparable. The body is able to produce spirit while the latter can command the former. The spirit will not exist without the body and vice versa. It is impossible for there to be a body without spirit or spirit without the body. A strong body produces a strong spirit, whereas a weak body contains a declined spirit. The so-called "the body represents the spirit", "the spirit represents the body", "the body and the spirit cannot be divided into two", "the body is spirit and spirit is the body" or "the body and mind are a unity of one", all refer to the same dialectical materialist point of view that the body and spirit are a unity. It is based on this theory that in the treatment of a disease, Chinese medicine pays great attention to the unity of body and mind or spirit and puts emphasis on the importance of treating psychological or mental problems prior to physical troubles, that is, psychological disturbances should be adjusted first.

4. The theory that the heart is in charge of the mental activities

Ancient people experienced in their life that under different spiritual states, the heart activities were different. When one was calm, the heart beat stably, but when one was excited, it beat faster. From these phenomena, they assumed that psychological activities were the heart's function and the heart was the organ performing psychological activities. In the earliest medical work extant in China, *The Yellow Emperor's Internal Classic*, the theories of all schools at the time were adopted and summed up into the theory that "the heart is in charge of mental activities." In the chapter "The Functions of Viscera" of the book *Plain Questions*, it is pointed out that " the heart is the monarch organ where mental activities take place." The chapter "Explanation to Five Kinds of Qi" records: "The heart houses the spirit." In another chapter, "Pathogenic Factors to the Body", it is further stated that "the heart is the master of all the viscera and the place where the spirit lives. When it is strong, the disease cannot find a way there. If a disease manages to lodge there, then the heart will be affected, the spirit will leave and death will ensue."

In TCM, the heart is compared to the monarch, which means it is not only the commander and core of all the viscera and all vital activities in the human body, but also the commander and core of human psychological activities. As the famous ancient physician Zhang Jiebin put it: "Soul, vigour, desire, will, worry, anxiety and the like are all spirit. In one word, spirit is kept in the heart. All emotions are under the command of the heart and so the heart is the spirit of the whole body." It can be inferred from this that the so-called "heart" in TCM, apart from the heart proper and its functions, also refers to thinking, feeling, will, imagination and psychological activities of various kinds occurring in the human brain.

It is just on the basis of the theory that the heart is in charge of mental activities that TCM advocates such psychotherapeutic methods as "relieving psychogenic factors", "mental tranquilization" or "calming the spirit and emotions".

5. The viscera-state and five-emotion theory

In TCM "viscera" refers to the solid internal viscera in the human body; "state" refers to the phenomena or external manifestations of the viscera. In TCM the condition of viscera mainly is determined by observing their external manifestations, that is, to visulize the state of internal organs by observing the external manifestations. This is the chief concern of the theory.

The TCM viscera-state theory has two characteristics. First, emphasis is put on the concept of a unified physiopsychic relationship between visceral condition and five emotions, that is, the five solid viscera produce five emotions. In other words, the five emotions are the external manifestations of the visceral activities. As "Explanation of Five Kinds of Qi", a chapter in *Plain Questions*, puts it: "The heart houses the spirit, the lung houses the soul, the liver houses mood, the spleen houses idea and the kidney houses will." Second, it is emphasized that when a solid internal organ is out of order, the manifestations related to the organ will become abnormal accordingly. As stated in "On Spirit", a chapter in *Miraculous Pivot*, "Heart palpitation due to fright and anxiety will hurt the spirit; and if the spirit is hurt, fright and terror will occur by themselves"; "Excessive joy of the lung will impair the soul, thereby a man becomes mad"; "Too much sorrow or grief causes impairment to mood, which may lead to madness and confusion." ⋯ TCM psychologists believe that the spirit, soul, mood, idea and will referred to in *The Yellow Emperor's Internal Classic* are indeed five different mental states, including the complicated changes of psychological activities such as the consciousness, memory, thinking, imagination and will. It is on the basis of this viscera-state and five-emotion theory that from the external manifestations the state of the internal organs can be inferred, and the configuration and spirit are a unity that TCM psychotherapy guides its clinical treatment.

6. The brain marrow theory

It has been held in TCM since ancient times that human psychological activities are closely related with the brain. In the medical book *The Yellow Emperor's Internal Classic* that was written 2 000 years ago, it was understood that the brain and spinal cord have the functions of producing psychological activities like vision and thinking and it is clearly stated there that the brain has a direct action on the psychological activities, normal or abnormal. For example, it is stated in "On the Seas in the Human Body", a chapter in *Miraculous Pivot*: "The brain is the sea of marrow⋯; if the brain is sufficient, a man feels robust and agile; if it is insufficient, a man may have dizziness, tinnitus, lassitude in the legs, blurred vision, slackness and sleepiness." It is further pointed out in "On Essence of Sphygmology", a chapter in the book *Plain Questions*, that "A man with spirit is able to see everything, to tell white from black, to tell a long thing from a short one; if a man cannot tell the difference between long and short, white and black, he lacks spirit⋯. The head is the residence of spirit. If a man cannot hold up his head and see far, he will soon lose his spirit." The above statements point out that human psychological activities, or spirit and thinking, are the products of the brain. If the brain is well developed, the psychological activities will be normal; whereas if the brain is not well developed or the brain marrow is insufficient, then psychological activities will be abnormal. That is why psychologists often treat abnormality of psychological activities by tonifying the brain and promoting the production of spinal marrow in clinical practice.

The Causes of Psychological Disturbance in Diabetics

1. Born weak diathesis

TCM holds that the main cause of diabetes is a weak diathesis with functional insufficiency of viscera. Improper diet, overstrain and excessive sexual activities also play important parts because they overly consume Yin and energy resulting in Yin deficiency and excessive heat, which cause impairment to the lung, stomach and kidney. According to the theories that body and spirit are a unity and five viscera produce five emotions, the weak diathesis and functional insufficiency of the five viscera will surely affect the emotions and psychological activities related to a certain internal organ to render the patient abnormal in such psychological activities as feelings, thinking, character, speech and senses.

Western medicine holds that diabetes has, etiologically, a genetic predisposition and is related to hypoimmunity. It is owing to the gene defect or gene mutation along with hypoimmunity that diabetes is likely to develop. Once diabetes develops, the patient will show some psychological and emotional abnormalities as well as physical changes because the patient is weak in constitution and has a poor body resistance, so his ability of stress to foreign stimuli is low and his psychological capacity is insufficient.

2. Impairment due to seven emotions

It is believed in TCM that although there are various causes of diabetes, some are the key ones. Just as the saying goes that "There are thousands of diseases, but their causes can be assorted to no more than three aspects." They are the six pathogenic climatic conditions, seven persistent and violent emotions, and improper diet and overstrain. An important cause of susceptibility to psychological abnormality in diabetics is emotional disturbance.

In the course of understanding things around oneself or contact with other people, one is never indifferent to people and things but always displays some feelings or emotions which can be summed up as seven: joy, anger, melancholy, anxiety, sorrow, fear and terror. Within the normal range, the emotions do not have so much influence on human health as to cause diseases, but when the emotions from the internal or environmental stimuli are too violent, or the stimuli are too strong and persistent for a long period to exceed the normal range, they will become pathogenic factors to cause derangement of Qi, blood, Yin and Yang, obstruction in channels and collaterals, disorder of visceral functions, and in the end lead to different kinds of pathological changes as well as corresponding abnormal emotional activities and psychological changes such as wild joy, melancholy, anxiety, sorrow, fear and terror.

As far as diabetics are concerned, because of genetic factors and immunological inadequacy, they are born weak in constitution and their visceral functions are insufficienct. As a result, their psychological bearing capacity and adaptive capacity to internal and external environmental stimuli are usually low. When such a diabetic patient is faced with such stress situations as an unexpected incident in life, sudden change of environment, or frustrated wishes, he tends to be unable to live with them and to make compromise with himself. As a result, he is likely to suffer psychological injury and abnormal psychological conflict to show varying degrees of abnormality in corresponding psychological sentiment.

The Characteristics of Psychological Disturbance of Diabetics

1. Emotional abnormality

(1) Excessive worry: Many diabetic patients burden themselves with excessive worries after they have gotten the disease. Instead of finding out how to cure his disease, such a patient may worry all day long about what would happen if his disease could not be cured, what he should do about the complications if they

developed, and what influence his disease would have on his work, study, future, family, etc. These thoughts often lead the patient into frustration and melancholy, and this psychological state is more likely to aggravate it other than help him in the treatment of the disease.

(2) Vexation and restlessness: Some diabetics fail to have a correct understanding of the chronic nature of the disease, so they often lack patience with their treatment but go to great lengths to look for a "miraculous doctor" and hope he could prescribe some "wonder drugs" to cure them of their disease in a short period of time. Once the treatment is not satisfactory in a short period, or their disease has relapses or complications develop, they become upset, disturbed, anxious and agitated or even develop insomnia at night, which is more harmful to the recovery.

(3) Nervousness and fright: Some diabetics are nervous about their disease, often misunderstanding it as an incurable disease. Especially when they hear that someone has died of ketoacidosis, or has been subjected to amputation due to gangrene in the lower limbs, or becomes blind as a result of bleeding in the optical fundus, they grow so nervous and frightened that they are in a constant state of anxiety, and thus feel depressed, lose their appetite, sleep poorly with many nightmares and become emaciated day by day. This horrified psychological state can only worsen the disease rather than help it.

(4) Irritability and quick anger: Some patients become so nervous when they know what they have gotten that they tend to lose their temper very easily and are very irritable to the things around and environment. They often become angry at trifles. They lack self control and patience. Anything, including study or work, that is not satisfactory will make them impetuous and angry. It is common in clinic that this kind of patient does not follow the physician's order for a systematic treatment. Whenever there is a relapse in their condition, they blame their doctors for their skill or blame their family for inconsiderate care of them. As a result, their condition is always changeable and progressive due

to their irritable psychological state.

(5) Sadness and susceptibility to tears: Some patients feel sorrowful when they know what they have gotten, especially when complications occur such as nephropathic uremia, bleeding in the optical fundus due to retinopathy, or amputation of a leg due to gangrene. They lose confidence in overcoming the disease, look worried, depressed and dejected. They often weep secretly, are sometimes so disheartened, despaired and pessimistic that they give up the desire to live and may even commit suicide. For such patients at the same time of pharmacotherapy, careful psychotherapy should be given to regulate the abnormal psychological state, so that satisfactory therapeutic effects may be achieved.

2. Abnormal disposition

Disposition is the psychological attributes which are fairly stable and of key importance and are embodied in an individual's attitude towards reality and in the manner of his behavior. Everybody has his own character traits, some of which are positive and some negative. When one is afflicted by a disease, his character may be changed. The same is true of diabetic patients who exhibit two kinds of changes in psychology and character. One kind of change is manifested as active or optimistic psychology and character. Those with this change are cheerful, bright, optimistic and frank. Neither do they lower their guard and become careless about their condition nor do they become nervous. They have a correct and scientific attitude to their disease and full confidence in overcoming it. They try to be emotionally stable and even if complications develop, they are able to cope with them. They are not sad and passive, but cooperate well with doctors and nurses in the treatment of their disease, so their condition is more likely to be improved and stablized instead of worsening. On the contrary, the other kind of change is manifested as passive psychology and character. Patients with this kind of change are depressed, irritable, uncommunicative, eccentric and introversive. At the beginning of their disease, they often lack the necessary vigilance and attention, but when their condition becomes worse or complications develop, they become excessively nervous. Worse still, they don't have a correct understanding of and scientific attitude to the disease, so that most of them are emotionally unstable, overly anxious, restless, irritable, sad and melancholic. They tend to lose confidence in overcoming the disease, and often fail to cooperate with doctors and nurses in their treatment, so their disease is often difficult to control but easy to aggravate. The abnormal psychology and character frequently seen in diabetics can be classified into the following types:

(1) Pessimistic type: This kind of patients are introversive in character. They are uncommunicative, eccentric and sorrowful. If their condition turns unfavourable or complications develop, they are very likely to become upset, pessimistic and disappointed, losing the confidence in the treatment of the disease, and tend to be unwilling to cooperate with doctors and nurses. They may even come up with the thought of committing suicide. Consequently, their condition is more often than not further aggravated. The common clinical features are vexation, palpitation, insomnia, frequent startling, dreaminess, poor appetite, dull look in the eyes, grief and tendency to weep. In severe cases, the patient does not eat and sleep at all.

(2) Easily enraged type: Such patients have an irascible temperament and are easily excited. They are poor in self-control, not calm when something happens, irritable and easily become angry when anything is not satisfactory. They lack patience for the treatment and often fail to cooperate with doctors and nurses during treatment. The common clinical features are irascibility, insomnia, dreaminess, dysphoria with feverish sensation in the chest, palms and soles, dry throat, bitter mouth, oppressed feeling in the chest, pain in the hypochondria, dizziness, and fullness of head. The patient's condition always becomes worse after a spell of anger.

(3) Worrying type: Such patients are overcautious and sentimental in everyday life. They usually can not stand any pessimal stimulation. They are happy whenever the treatment is effective

or their condition turns favourable, but whenever there is a relapse or aggravation in their condition, they become full of worries and cannot come to terms with themselves and their condition. The clinical features are troubled thoughts, worries, a mournful contenance, oppressed feeling in the chest, shortness of breath, frequent sighing, insomnia, dreaminess, and poor appetite.

(4) Qi-stagnation type: The patient is timid, mistrustful and introversive by nature. He never talks out his mind when faced with any problem but always remains in the blues and cannot walk out of his mood. The typical clinical features are a disturbed mind, an oppressed feeling in the chest, distending pain in the hypochondria with a pain difficult to locate, eructation and poor appetite. He is not confident in the recovery of his disease and is unable to cooperate with the doctors during his treatment. Consequently, his condition is difficult to be controlled.

Common Psychotherapy Methods in the Treatment of Diabetes

1. Verbal enlightening

This method is also known as speech enlightening and behaviour induction treatment, being the most basic and most commonly used method of psychotherapy. It refers to the speech and behaviour of the doctors in the course of diagnosis and treatment of a patient's disease, with which doctors try to influence the patient's psychology to adjust the patient's abnormal psychology and treat his disease. There are some very brilliant expositions on the gist of this method in "Biography of the Master", a chapter in *Miraculous Pivot*. It says: "As far as the human nature is concerned, there is no one who does not detest death and enjoy life. If he is informed about what is harmful to life and what is beneficial, helped to understand what should be done and what causes pain to him, even the ignoramus will follow your advice."

To sum up, the method includes the following four aspects: ① To explain to the patient the nature, pathogenic factors, the harm to the body, and common complications of diabetes so as to help him pay attention to the disease and have a correct objective understanding of it. ②To increase the patient's confidence in subduing his disease by patiently telling him that if he is given timely treatment, cooperates with doctors, takes medicine according to the doctor's orders, the prognosis will be good. ③ To tell the patient the ways of keeping in good health, such as "giving up sex, avoiding anger, going on a diet, leading a regular life, and keeping off heresy". ④ At the same time of psychotherapy, importance should be attached to physical and psychological treatment and nursing so as to help the patient feel free from nervousness, worry, fright and passive attitude. This method is easy for the patient to accept and so the effects are desirable.

2. Diverting attention

The psychotherapy of diverting attention means the patient's attention to his disease is diverted to other things. Some patients are very nervous when the diagnosis of their disease is established as diabetes, and they concentrate their thoughts on diabetes, worrying all the time that the disease would get worse or could not be cured. They imagine so much around their disease that they are deeply troubled by the worries. When they hear that some diabetic suffers from diabetic gangrene or bleeding in the optical fundus they are so scared that they grow more nervous and are in a constant state of anxiety. Even worse, some patients are unable to go into sleep at all. When their disease is complicated by pathological changes in peripheral nerves which give rise to numbness and aching in the limbs, some patients usually suspect that they have got diabetic gangrene that will lead to amputation of a limb. Thereafter, they focus their attention on the complication and become all the more sensitive to the numbness and aching in the limb. The suspicion and oversensitivity greatly interfere with their work or study and render the treatment ineffective. For this kind of patients, speech induction should be conducted to persuade and influence patients so as to divert the patient's attention, which may have a therapeutic effect that simple pharmacotherapy can not produce, or even pharmacotherapy is unnecessary at all.

It is pointed out in "On Treatment of Disease with Grafting Spirit and Altering Qi in Witchcraft" of the book *Plain Questions* that in the antiquity, the treatment of a disease was conducted purely through "grafting spirit and altering Qi". Grafting spirit refers to deverting or transferring the patient's spirit, will, worry and attention. Altering Qi refers to diverting the patient's attention and promoting the flow of Qi and blood to alter and regulate the functional activities of Qi and thus to relieve or eliminate the disease. "Grafting spirit and altering Qi" is in fact a psychotherapy by means of diverting the patient's attention.

The application of this method can be found in case records of famous ancient doctors. For example, Ye Tianshi (1667-1746) recorded in his book *A Guide to Clinical Practice With Medical Records* how he succeeded in curing a case of diabetes by using the method of diverting attention: Once a diabetic patient was referred to him for treatment. He found that the patient was so nervous that he worried about his disease all the time and suspected his condition would turn worse. As a result, he failed to respond to medical treatment. Dr. Ye contemplated that if the patient could divert his attention by growing flowers and bamboo, the pharmacotherapy would work; otherwise, if the patient worried about his condition all day long, no medicine would work. Ye's train of thought was that the cure of the disease "lies in the patient's alteration of temperament and disposition", that is, to divert the patient's attention to make him relaxed and thereby cure his disease.

3. Emotion-overcome-emotion method

This method can be interpreted as overpowering one emotion by another. The method is based on the principle of interrelations of the five evolusive elements. In the treatment with this method, man-made emotions are used to stimulate and affect the patient so that his abnormal psychological activities can be normalized and thus the patient's condition can be improved. According to TCM theories, the seven emotional changes—joy, anger, melancholy, anxiety, sorrow, fear and terror—are not only one of the major pathogenic factors, but are also effective measures in the prevention and treatment of diseases. It has been proved by clinical practice that diseases resulting from the disturbace of the seven emotions can be treated by emotion-overcome-emotion psychotherapy with satisfactory clinical effects.

In "Grand Discussion On the Concept of Yin and Yang", a chapter of *Plain Questions* there is such exposition: "Anger tends to affect the liver but sorrow can check anger; overjoy affects the heart but fear can check it; anxiety affects the spleen but anger can check it; melancholy affects the lung, but joy can check it; fear affects the kidney but anxiety can check it." According to this principle, in our clinical practice, we often treat diseases, e. g. diabetes, caused by emotional disturbances with emotion-overcome-emotion psychotherapy in addition to pharmacotherapy. For diabetes due to affection of the liver by anger, sorrow can be used to overcome anger; for diabetes due to affection of the heart by overjoy, fear can be used to overcome overjoy; if it is due to affection of the spleen by anxiety, anger is used; if due to affection of the lung by sorrow, joy is used; and if due to affection of the kidney by fear, anxiety can be used. These are the concrete application of emotion-overcome-emotion psychotherapy. The five viscera of the human body generate five emotions as anger, joy, anxiety, sorrow and fear, which are related respectively to the five viscera and interpromote or check one another in the same way as the five evolusive elements do. On one hand, the five emotions— anger (liver-wood), joy (heart-fire), anxiety (spleen-earth), sorrow (lung-metal) and fear (kidney-water)—interpromote each other, each promoting or producing the subsequent one in the listed sequence; on the other hand, they interact to restrain or check one another in the following sequence: wood checks earth, which checks water, which checks fire, which checks metal, which checks wood, that is, anger (liver-wood) can check excessive anxiety (spleen-earth), anxiety can check excessive fear (kidney-water), and fear, joy (heart-fire), sorrow (lung-metal), anger

33

(liver-wood) can check the subsequent one in turn. In light of this principle and by studying the emotional activities of a diabetic patient, a corresponding emotion-overcome-emotion method can be applied, which often brings about a very remarkable effect that pharmacotherapy alone cannot achieve.

4. Mental tranquilization

This method is also known as "calming down the spirit and emotions", which is a psychotherapy laying emphasis on keeping the spirit inside (keeping a sound mind). In TCM, great importance has always been attached to the positive effect of keeping the spirit inside in the prevention and treatment of diseases. It was put forward in *The Yellow Emperor's Internal Classic* that "The spirit is stored when one is calm but dies out when one is impetuous." And it was also stated that "If one is indifferent to fame and gain and disillusioned with the mortal world, the genuine Qi will be with him; when one keeps the spirit inside, how can diseases come about?" These statements emphasize that if one can keep a peaceful mind, he will seldom catch a disease and can enjoy a long healthy life. Even if he is affected by a disease, it is easy to be cured and the restoration of health is not difficult. This is because "The spirit is kept inside". On the contrary, if one is impetuous, he is susceptible to diseases, which tend to be difficult to cure. Just as stated in Essential Therapies, a chapter in *Plain Questions*, "When everyone keeps his Qi settled and himself quiet and calm, the pathogenic factors will die off. This is the essence of medicine." It is implied in these statements that the psychotherapy of calming down the emotions to tranquilize the mind is of great importance in the prevention and treatment of diseases.

The pathogenesis of diabetes is chiefly due to a deficiency of Liver Yin and Kidney Yin resulting in excessive dryness-heat in the lung and stomach, deficiency of Yin and body fluid, and development of pathogenic fire of deficiency type in the interior. Apart from the symptoms of polydipsia, polyphagia, polyuria, and emaciation, the patient often manifests impatience, worry, irritability and restlessness. Pharmacotherapy alone usually does not have satisfactory effects, but when it is combined with such psychotherapy methods as calming down emotions to tranquilize the mind and clearing the mind of all worries to rest quietly, desirable effects can always be achieved. As for the concrete measures of these methods, a brilliant exposition was made in *A New Book on How to Help Your Parents to Preserve Health and Prolong Their Lives* written in the Yuan Dynasty (1271-1368 AD): "Those who are good at caring for life should, first, not talk much so as to conserve the internal Qi; second, give up lust to conserve the promordial-Qi; third, avoid spicy and salty food to tonify the blood; fourth, often swallow the saliva to nourish the viscera; fifth, never get angry to protect the Liver Qi; sixth, pay attention to diet to protect the Stomach Qi; and seventh, be free from anxiety and worries to spare the Heart Qi. Man develops from Qi and Qi is kept by the spirit. If one pays attention to maintain Qi well and keep the spirit intact, he will attain the true Way.

5. Desirability fancy

Also known as imagining cheerful mood method, it is a psychotherapy with which the patient is inspired through speech induction to be cheerful and happy so that he will build up confidence in overcoming his disease. Usually the mood and spirits, good or bad, of a person have much to do with the generation, development and changes of diseases. Generally, when one is happy and cheerful, he feels satisfactory about whatever he does. If he is ill, it is easy for him to recover. Contrarily, when one is sorrowful, he often weeps, feels disheartened and becomes pessimistic and despairing. Everything in the world seems gloomy to him. In this mood it is easy for him to catch diseases but difficult for his diseases to be cured, or even worse, the disease is likely to deteriorate. The following is stated in *Jingyue's Complete Works*: "When one is ill due to a melancholic mood, no treatment is effective unless the patient regains ease of mind and his wishes come true."

Therefore, many physicians in ancient times believed that only when the patient was cheerful and happy, had ease of mind, and was perfectly content, could the medicine be effective for his disease; otherwise, no matter how much medicine he took, there would be little effect. In our treatment of diabetes, we attach great importance to psychological treatment that can render the patient cheerful and happy. We cite as many examples as possible who have recovered from the disease or whose conditions have distinctly improved. We also go out of our way to explain to the patient that as long as the treatment is systematic and scientific, the complications can be prevented. This makes patients have ease of mind and free their minds of worries so they can build up confidence in curing their disease. On the basis of psychotherapy, pharmacotherapy is given and satisfactory result can be achieved in most cases.

6. Regulating Qi through physical and breathing exercise

This method is also called treatment with Qigong expiration and inspiration or with regulation of mental faculties to rest the mind. It is a psychotherapy which emphasizes psychosomatic treatment and whose theoretic core is adjustment of body posture, regulation of respiration and regulation of mental activities. TCM has emphasized the important role of physical and breathing exercises in psychotherapy since ancient times. Among the medical books copied on silk unearthed in 1973 from the tombs of the Han Dynasty at Mawangdui in Changsha, there is a special treatise on disease prevention and treatment by means of physical and breathing exercises, to which some drawings of exercises are attached. According to Biography of Hua Tuo in *The History of Three Kingdoms*, the famous doctor Hua Tuo was very good at treating diseases and caring for life with physical and breathing exercises. He said: "The human body should be exercised but not exhausted to the utmost. Through exercise the food eaten is well digested and blood circulation is promoted so that one will not be afflicted with diseases just as a moving door pivot never decays." Hua Tuo also devised a set of physical fitness exercises "Five Mimic-animal Boxing".

From the modern point of view, the physical and breathing exercises are a psychosomatic therapy with Qigong exercises as the principal substance. The concrete requirements of the exercises can be summed up as three stages or three essentials: adjustment of posture, regulation of respiration and regulation of mental activities. By adjustment of the body posture, it is meant that the body is made relaxed naturally to induce the relaxation of the mind. By regulation of respiration, it is meant that the respiration is regulated by thought to make one's thought and ideas unitary so that one can banish distracting thoughts from the mind, sit still and achieve mental calmness. By regulation of mental activities, it is meant to regulate the mental state so that one can sit still, achieve mental calmness, concentrate ideas, thoughts and imagination on a certain part inside the human body (e.g. Dantian) or on a certain object or thing outside the body (e.g. counting numbers or listening to one's own breathing). It is also called mind concentration and is the critical stage to successful physical and breathing exercises. Although the adjustment of body posture, regulation of respiration and regulation of mental acitivities are an organic entity, the latter plays a leading role.

The substantial content of physical and breathing exercises are Qigong, whose mechanism of action in the treatment of diabetes will be discussed in a special chapter later on.

Attaching Importance to Psychological Care for Diabetics

1. Principles for psychological care

(1) Absolute sincerity and honesty. Doctors and nurses should treat diabetic patients with sincere and deep feelings in much the same way that they treat their own family members, being considerate all the time and showing the utmost solicitude, because when one is sick, he tends to feel lonely, depressed, worried and sad, and has an urgent need for warm care from his family, relatives and especially from medical workers. Every doctor and nurse should, therefore, treat diabetic patients enthusiastically, show-

ing concern, understanding and sympathy for them. Only in this way can they enjoy the trust of their patients, who will in turn build up the confidence to overcome the disease and cooperate well with medical workers during their treatment.

(2) Treat all patients equally without discrimination. The famous ancient doctor Sun Simiao emphsized in his work, *Essential Prescriptions Worth A Thousand Gold* : "A great doctor who is to practice medicine must make up his mind to devote himself to the trade, be free from any desire to make demands from his patients but should first of all have great pity and sympathy for his patients and pledge to relieve the sufferings of any one who comes to him. When a patient comes to him for help, he is not to identify the patient as rich or poor, noble or humble. No matter whether his patients are old or young, ugly or pretty, closely or far related to him, amicable or hostile, Chinese or alien, foolish or wise, he is to treat them all equally and indiscriminately like kinsfolk." What Sun Simiao said should be followed by all doctors and nurses. To medical workers, patients can only be divided into emergent or ordinary, mild or severe, but not poor or rich, noble or humble.

(3) Treatment according to individual differences: As *The Yellow Emperor's Internal Classic* has put it, "People are born different; some are strong in character, others are gentle; some are of weak build, others are of strong build; some are tall, others are short; some are men and others are women." Owing to differences in heredity, environment, education, family background, profession, sex, age, financial condition, knowledge, experience, emotional tendency, will, need, interests, ability, temperament, disposition, and also the characteristics and duration of the disease, the patient's psychological states are quite different. In the course of psychological care, therefore, different methods should be employed for different patients, and the care should be both patient and meticulous. Apart from positive guidance and deep feeling to affect all patients, different methods must be adopted to solve different problems of different individuals. The

psychological care cannot follow one single pattern and empty talk should be avoided so that the care is to the heart of every patient to achieve the best nursing result.

2. Methods of psychological care

(1) Heart-to-heart talk: Become close to the patient by chatting and talking about everyday matters with him or her so as to know the characteristics of the patient's psychological activities and psychological state, help him or her to eliminate the passive ideas and build up a good psychological state and have the patient mentally prepared to cure his disease.

(2) Explanation: In view of the patient's worries, tell him about the related medical knowledge to help him rid his mind of all the worries and to build up confidence in overcoming his disease.

(3) Enlightening the patient by reasoning: By telling him the emotional causes of the disease, the patient is made to realize the emotional disturbance of "uncontrolled excessive joy and anger" is a most important cause of all diseases, while "neutralizing joy and anger" and "controlled joy and anger" is the basis of good health and longevity. On this basis the patient is enlightened to consciously avoid anger and control his emotions.

(4) Preaching medical knowledge: To preach medical knowledge to the patient, explain the causes, pathogenesis and changes of his disease, and the ways of self-care so that the patient will know how to prevent and treat the disease, how to have self-care, and how to cooperate well with medical workers to improve the therapeutic effects.

(5) Avoiding further emotional irritation: In the course of diagnosis and treatment, medical workers should try their best to protect the patient from further psychological and social irritation, which, undoubtedly, is adverse to the patient's condition.

Dietotherapy to Diabetes

The Concept of Dietotherapy

Dietotherapy refers to the ways in which one can conserve his health to prevent diseases through proper diet and treat diseases with proper diet. It is a means and measure to influence the body functions and to keep fit or cure a disease by taking in different food. Food is the important material basis for treating diseases and restoring health; it has not only therapeutic effect on a patient's organs but also a many-sided overall influence on the whole body.

Chinese dietotherapy has a long history and has accumulated rich experience in treating diseases by proper dieting. *The Dietetic Materia Medica* compiled in the Tang Dynasty noted the functions of food in the prevention and treatment of diseases, described the flavour, property and health-conserving efficacy of many kinds of food. Take the description of the lotus root in the book for example. It is "cold in property, good at invigorating the middle Jiao, nourishing the vitality, increasing strength and eliminating all diseases. One becomes agile and cold-resistant, does not easily feel hungry and enjoys longevity if it is taken for a long time." Wax gourd is decribed as "cold in property, chiefly indicated for water retention in the lower abdomen, and also good for urine problems and diabetes." On the importance of dietotherapy, *Prescriptions Worth a Thousand Gold for Emergencies* points out that "The foundation of a good health is the knowledge of food. If one does not know what is proper for food, he cannot live well." It is mentioned in *Plain Questions* that "Before making a diagnosis, questions about the dieting habit and daily life must be asked." It is also recorded in *General Treatise on Causes and Symptoms of Diseases* that diabetics should eat wheat bran, pear, water chestnut, Chinese yam and spiral-shelled food. Now it has been proved that limited amount of food of wheat bran and Chinese yam is good for diabetics.

The development of modern medicine has further proved that a proper diet for a diabetic can increase the patient's body resistance, promote the restoration of the metabolic function of the tissues and reasonably control the generation and development of complications. The diet for diabetic patients should be a well-balanced one with all the necessary nutrients in good proportions. A good variety of food is an essential condition for obtaining all the necessary nutrients. The diet should be well balanced between the staple food and the non-staple, between the coarse food grains and the fine ones, between meat and vegetables, and must be taken at strictly planned times and in limited amount. Only in this way can the diet be beneficial to the recovery of diabetes and improvement of constitution.

The Aim of Dietotherapy

Dietotherapy is one of the essential therapies for diabetes and an important therapeutic method. Dietotherapy does not mean a blind reduction of food intake, but has its purposes. The first aim of dietotherapy for diabetes is to take in the minimum amount of carbohydrates to maintain the normal requirements of the body, relieve the burden of islet β-cells, correct the metabolic disturbance, ameliorate symptoms, so that the glucose in blood and urine and blood-lipid can be kept at a normal or roughly normal level to prevent or delay the generation and development of complications. Another aim of dietotherapy is to maintain a normal body weight by reducing the weight in fat patients and increaseing body weight in emaciated patients. In the practice of dietotherapy, practical and realistic dietary recipes well balanced in nutrition should be formulated to improve the nutritional condition of the body and increase body resistance. *The Golden Chamber of Medicine* has pointed out: "The food taken may be beneficial to a disease or harmful to the body. If it is beneficial to the disease, then it is good to health; if harmful to the body, it will bring about diseases." To make up deficiency in the body with food so that body resistance can be restored to prevent the body from affection of diseases and maintain health, this is the goal that dietotherapy should try to attain.

The Basic Principles of Dietotherapy

Diagnosis and treatment based on an overall analysis of symptoms and signs, the cause, nature and location of the illness and the patient's physical condition in the light of the basic theories of TCM is not only a basic principle in TCM therapeutics, but also a basic principle in dietotherapy.

Different individuals are endowed with different diatheses, constitutions, characters and personal likings. Even in a same individual, there are differences in the constitutional condition and functional state of Qi and blood in different stages of life, so when dietotherapy is to be given, full consideration must be taken in these aspects so as to adopt a most appropriate dietary plan. For people of different sex, age, constitution, etc., the diet should be different. For example, in fat people, there tends to be more phlegm and dampness, so it is preferable for them to have more light and phlegm-dissolving food while in emaciated people, there tends to be a deficiency of Yin, blood and body fluid, so they should have more food which nourishes Yin and promotes the production of body fluid.

Moreover, the physiological functions of people vary with seasonal and climatic changes, which should, therefore, also be taken into account in the course of dietotherapy. Spring is a season in which everything begins to grow and Yang Qi also begins to develop, so it is not suitable for people to have much greasy and spicy food lest this will lead to leakage of Yang Qi out of the body. More vegetables and food made from bean products should be included in the diet. In summer, the climate is hot and there are more rains, the functions of the spleen and stomach are often hampered by heat and dampness to affect the appetite. If one indulges himself in too much cold and raw food or the food is not clean, diarrhea and dysentery are likely to happen. So in summer, people are encouraged to have food which is light or non-greasy, sweet and cold in property, and advantageous to clearing away heat, such as mung bean tea and rice porridge with lotus leaf. In autumn, cool wind begins to blow, very dry air prevails and cold dew and frost begin to form. One is apt to be affected by cold in the early morning and late evening to give rise to cough or relapse of bronchitis. Food such as turnip (or raddish), apricot kernel, rice porridge with coix seed should be often had to clear away heat from the lung, lower the Lung Qi and dissolve phlegm. In winter the weather is cold and the ground is frozen. In this season, one is very likely to be affected by cold pathogens. For prevention, one should have hot porridge in the morning and choose food of warm or hot property to fight against cold, but it is unwise to have too much rich and heavy food lest it should lead to accumulation of dampness and generation of phlegm. In one word, the diabetic patients should have the right food with the changes of seasons to meet the body's needs.

A proper dietary plan should be worked out for a diabetic patient according to his or her constitution, seasonal climatic changes, and the type of his or her diabetes. Diabetes due to excessive heat in the lung and excessive heart-fire is often a complication of a heat-syndrome, so the principle of treatment is clearing away heat and promoting production of body fluid because when heat is removed and there is enough body fluid, the diabetes will heal subsequently. The food for such a patient should be of neutral or slightly cold property, and the amount of cold-natured food can be decided in view of the severity of heat syndrome. The diet should be light. Greasy, hot, roasted and deep-fried food should be avoided, or taken in small amount, for they promote generation of heat and fire. For diabetics with sweet urine, sweet food is not appropriate and food made from cereals, potato and sweet potato should be taken in strictly limited amount. In the case of diabetes with dysfunction of stomach and spleen marked by lack of appetite, indigestion and abdominal distention, the patient should have more soup and porridge instead of solid food, and frequent small meals to protect the Stomach Qi. If the patient suffers from polyphagia and bulimia, he usually cannot stand the reduction of food intake, in which case, more food prepared from coarse grains should be given instead of that made from fine ones, and more low-calorie, large-bulk food should be given. Emaciated patients should increase the intake of calories and proteins but the amount should be strictly controlled. On the contrary, obese patients should decrease the intake of calories. The minimum nutritional requirements, however, should be guaranteed and the intake of protein should not be too low. The patient should eat lean meat but not greasy food such as fat meat and deep-fried food. The food should be cooked with as little oil as possible. It is very important for the patient to have a good control of his appetite and a meal should not consist of many things. Even if a kind of food subserves a patient's condition, it should not be taken excessively. If taken too much at a time, the food is likely to hurt the spleen and stomach and to cause more damage than benefit.

The Control of Total Calorie Intake

Carbohydrates, fats and proteins are oxidized in the human body to provide it with heat. The total calorie intake should be determined according to a patient's standard body weight, living condition, labour intensity and nature of the work. The calories needed per kilogram of body weight per day is: adult at rest: 104.6-122.5J (25-30cal); adult doing light physical work:

122.5-146.4J (30-35cal); adult doing moderate physical work: 146.4-167.4J (35-40cal); adult doing heavy work: 167.4J (40cal).

Here below are several formulae for calculating the standard body weight:

1. Height (cm) − 105 = standard body weight (kg)
2. [Height(cm) − 100] × 0.9 = standard body weight (kg)
3. $\text{Height(cm)} - 100 - \frac{\text{Height(cm)} - 150}{4}$ = standard body weight(kg) for male

   $\text{Height(cm)} - 100 - \frac{\text{Height(cm)} - 150}{2}$ = standard body weight(kg) for female

In case the actual body weight is more than the standard, the total calorie intake should be deducted by 15% while 15% of the total calorie intake can be added if the actual body weight is less than the standard. For pregnant women, breast-feeding mothers, children in growth and development period, and those whose body weight is below the standard due to malnutrition or consumptive diseases, the total calorie intake can be increased by 10%-20%, and for notably emaciated diabetics, the total calorie intake in food can be further increased during the recovery stage.

The allocation of carbohydrate, fat and protein:

1. Protein

1-1.5g is needed per kilogram of body weight per day for an adult. The intake may be increased to 2-3g for pregnant women, children, breast-feeding mothers, those suffering from malnutrition or consumptive diseases, accounting for 20% of the total heat intake. Because of the increased gluconeogenesis in the body of diabetics, protein is consumed in large quantities. When diabetes is associated with diabetic renopathy, a great deal of protein is discharged with urine, so if the renal function allows, more protein should be taken in; and if the renal function is decreased, the intake of protein should be limited.

Such foods as soybean, fish, chicken, shrimp, lean meat, milk and egg contain plenty of protein. It is desirable that one third of the daily intake of protein should come from animal sources because animal protein contains abundant essential amino-acids which are the materials needed for the metabolism of protein in the nutrients for the human body.

2. Fat

Fat intake for an adult should be 1g per kilogram of body weight per day, which accounts for no more than 30%-35% of the total heat taken in. For obese patients with hyperlipoproteinemia or atherosclerosis, the intake of fat should be controlled under 30% of the total heat intake. For patients with hypercholesterolemia or type II hyperlipoproteinemia, the daily cholesterol intake should be kept under 300mg. They should have very little animal fats and viscera, egg yolk, roe, etc. in their diet and eat as little fried food as they can help. The food should be cooked in vegetable oil. For diabetics with normal blood-lipid value and without atherosclerosis, it is better for their fat intake to be of animal and vegetable sources in equal halves.

3. Carbohydrate

A diabetic can take in 200-300g of carbohydrate, which refers to the intake of sugar-containing food, including starches in the staple food. The staple food should not be kept at a too low level, for if the patient is semi-hungry, it is difficult for his condition to be controlled. Staple foods such as rice and wheat flour contain adequate carbohydrate, and are the main source of vegetable protein. They are important and indispensible nutrients in the human body and the most economic and rapid source for supplying calories and protein. If the body takes in too little carbohydrate, the energy supplying process will make use of fat and protein in the body. If the carbohydrate intake is less than 25g a day, the fat will be decomposed and more ketone bodies will be produced; and if insulin is not in abundance to make full use of the ketone bodies, ketoacidosis will develop.

Food fiber, a kind of polysaccharide which does not produce thermal energy, can be classified as soluble and non-soluble. The non-soluble food fiber, including cellulose, hemicellulose and lignin, can be found in the pericarpium of the seeds of cereals and beans and in the stalk and leaf of plants. The soluble food fiber, including pectin, algin and bean gel is found in fruits, vegetables, sea-tangle, laver and beans. The content of these components in common vegetables is 20%-60%, and about 10% in fruits and cereals. More fiber-rich composition in food can help improve hyperglycemia and reduce the dosage of insulin and oral hypoglycemic agents.

Fiber-rich food may slow down the absorption of sugar by the delay of gastric emptying, change of the time of intra-intestinal transportation and gel formed by soluble fibers in the intestines. Fiber-rich food may also promote the metabolism of glucose by reducing the secretion of intestinal hormones like gastric inhibitory polypetide (GIP) or glucagon, the stimulation to the β-cells, the release of insulin, and by increasing the sensitivity of peripheral insulin-receptors.

The Dietary Calculation and Diet Planning

1. Dietary calculation

(1) Work out the patient's standard body weight with the aid of the formulae for calculating standard body weight according to the patient's age, sex, and height.

(2) Work out the heat the patient requires daily according to his standard body weight.

(3) Work out the protein requirement (1.5g per kilogram of body weight per day). One gram of protein generates 16.75kJ of heat.

(4) Work out the fat requirement (1g per kilogram of body weight per day). One gram of fat produces 37.68kJ of heat.

(5) Deduct the amount of heat produced by protein and fat from the total of daily heat requirement and the remaining portion will be provided by carbohydrate. 1g of carbohydrate generates 16.75kJ.

The calculation can be demonstrated by the following example.

A female patient, 45 years old, 165cm, 62kg, holding a job of light physical labor. After calaculation, her standard body weight should be 60kg.
$$165 - 105 = 60 (kg)$$
Daily total heat requirement:
$$60 \times 126^* = 7560 (kJ)$$

(* It refers to 126kJ. An individual of normal body weight who does heavy physical labour needs 168kJ per kilo of body weight per day, who does moderate physical labour needs 147kJ per kilo of body weight per day, who does light physical labour needs 126kJ per kilo of body weight per day, and who is under bed rest needs 63-84kJ per kilo of body weight per day.)

Protein:
$$60 \times 1.5 = 90 (g)$$
$$90 \times 16.75 = 1507.5 (kJ)$$

Fat:
$$60 \times 1 = 60 (g)$$
$$60 \times 37.68 = 2260.8 (kJ)$$

Carbohydrate:
$$7560 - (1507.5 + 2260.8) = 3791.7 (kJ)$$
$$3791.7 \div 16.75 \approx 226 (g)$$

It can be seen from the calculation that the patient should take 90g of protein, 60g of fat, 226g of carbohydrate every day with a total heat of 7560kJ.

It is preferable for a diabetic patient to have a diet according to the food intake requirement and special emphasis should be laid on small frequent meals, which can prevent the pancreatic islets from being overburdened by too much dietary heat, so that the blood sugar will not fluctuate too much and hypoglycemic reaction can be avoided. When the patient's condition is stable, the daily food intake should also be fixed, but when the condition changes, the daily food intake should be regulated. If the condition progresses, the food intake should be strictly controlled and should be less than usual. If the patient does more physical work, 25-50 grams of staple food can be added. Flexibility in the control of food intake is helpful for the patient as long as the flexibility keeps to the principle that the food eaten must be in good balance with the physical activities. The amount of food eaten should vary with the increase and decrease in physical activities.

2. Dietary planning

Four tables listing the content of nutrients in various kinds of food are provided here below to help diabetic patients be familiar with the nutritive elements in various kinds of food and will serve as a guide for their dietary planning.

Tab. 3-1 Nutrient Content in Food of the Three Meals

Meals	Food	Average Type (g)	Obese Type (g)	Lean Type (g)
Breakfast	Porridge	75	55	100
	Boiled egg	40	50	40
	Vegetable (stir-fried)	a little	55	100
Lunch	Rice	125	70	135
	Beef	55	90	100
	Vegetable (Containing 3% of sugar)	200	300	300
	Oil	15	10	10
Supper	Rice or steamed bread	150	70	135
	Vegetable	200	300	300
	Lean pork	50	–	–
	Chicken	–	70	–
	Duck	–	–	100
	Oil	6	13	12
Daily Nutrients	Carbohydrates	270	162	288
	Fat	53	33	49
	Protein	60	59	82
Total heat (kJ)		7560	4940	8060

49

Tab. 3-2 Nutrient Content in Common Staple Food (per 100g)

Food	Protein (g)	Fat (g)	Sugar (g)
Rice	6.7	0.9	78
Flour(Refined)	9.1	0.9	76
Flour(standard)	10.1	1.7	74
Noodle	9.6	1.7	70
Steamed bread of refined flour	6.1	0.2	40.1
Steamed bread of standard flour	9.9	1.8	43

Tab. 3-3 Sugar Content in Common Vegetables (per 100g of edible parts)

Sugar content	Vegetables
1%	purple bolt, pumpkin, tender cattail stem, marrow, water cress
2%	celery, yellowish leek, pakchoi, fennel leaves, agar, spinadge, wax gourd, cucumber, snake melon, garden lettuce
3%	leek, green amaranth, rape cos lettuce, balsam pear, tomato, Chinese cabbage, pea pod, lady's bedstraw
4%	garlic sprouts, cabbage, cauliflower, sowthistle, radish leaves, mung bean sprouts, potherb mustard, egg plant, spring bamboo shoots, bur clover, water spinach, wild rice stem, cowpea, towel gourd sword bean, mushroom
5%	winter bamboo shoots, Tianjin radish, shallot, lentil, cowpea pod
6%	soybean sprouts, white turnip, green soybean sprouts, green Chinese onion, lotus root
7%	green turnip, onion, Chinese toon, sweetbell redpepper, coriander, Chinese yam
8%	yellow carrot, red turnip, taro, potato
9%	garlic bulb, fresh day lily, lidney bean, pea, garlic bolt, broad bean

Tab. 3-4 Nutrient Content in Everyday Protein-rich Food (per 100g)

Food	Protein (g)	Fat (g)	Sugar (g)
Lean pork	16.7	28.8	1.1
Pork liver	20.1	4.0	3.0
Lean beef	20.3	6.2	1.7
Lean mutton	21.2	0.4	0.2
Chicken	23	1.2	–
Duck	16.5	7.5	0.1
Goose	10.8	11.2	–
Yellow croaker	17.6	0.8	–
Ribbonfish	18.1	7.4	–
Grass carp	17.9	4.3	–
Silver carp	18.6	4.8	–
Common carp	17.3	5.1	–
Crucian carp	13.0	1.1	0.1
Ricefield eel	18.8	0.9	–
Freshwater shrimp	17.5	0.6	–
Egg	14.8	11.6	0.5
Duck's egg	13.0	14.7	1.0
Milk	3.1	3.5	6.0
Soybean milk	5.2	2.5	3.7
Dried bean curd	19.2	6.7	6.7
Bean curd	4.7	1.3	2.8
Peanut	26.2	39.2	22.1

Points for Attention in Dietotherapy

Dietotherapy is very important for diabetes and has a positive therapeutic effect. In order to make full use of dietotherapy and to obtain the expected object, attention must be paid to the following points.

1. Regular meals

The diet of diabetic patients should be planned in such a way that the daily total heat intake should be divided by three meals as 1/5 for breakfast, 2/5 for both lunch and supper, so as to avoid too much fluctuation of blood sugar due to irrational food intake.

As for insulin-dependent patients, the daily total heat intake should be divided by four meals, that is, they should have one more meal before going to bed so that a better coordination between food intake and action time of insulin injection can be achieved.

2. Control on both staple and non-staple food

In the dietary planning, it is not preferable only to limit the intake of staple food but not the non-staple food. Some patients have a strict budget for staple food but put no limit to non-staple food. It must be known that some non-staple food such as meat, egg, beans, peanut and cooking oil contains much fat which provides enormous amount of heat, and if a diabetic patient takes such food more than necessary, he will find it unfavourable for him to control his condition. The intake of vegetables containing more than 4% of sugar, e.g. Chinese yam, potato, lentil, white turnip, red turnip, taro, lotus root, mushroom and soybean, should also be restricted and a deduction of equal amount of staple food should be made in terms of sugar intake.

3. Proper control over intake of carbohydrate

Clinical experience has proved that it is not true that the less carbohydrate a diabetic takes, the better. A good number of diabetics have strictly limited their intake of carbohydrate but they still have suffered from ketosuria because fat metabolism in the body requires the participation of sufficient amount of carbohydrate and if the supply of carbohydrate is not enough, more fat will be decomposed, leading to incomplete oxidation of fat to form ketone bodies, which accumulate in the body and are excreted with urine.

4. Proper increase of the content of food fiber

Food fiber is a polysuccharine which does not generate thermal energy but can help both obese and emaciated patients decrease blood-lipid, lower the level of blood sugar after meals, improve glucose tolerance and reduce the consumption of insulin. Therefore, the amount of food fiber in a diabetic's diet should be increased. As for how to increase it, it is preferable to get it from natural food such as whole wheat flour, dry bean, and fresh vegetables.

5. Low-salt diet

Salt is indispensable to the human body and is the main source of sodium ions and chlorine ions in the human body. However, it should not be taken too much by the body, for when it enters the body, salt activates amylase and promotes the digestion of starch and absorption of glucose by the small intestines to raise the level of blood sugar after meals. Salt intake should be kept under 10 grams a day, equal to about 4 000mg of sodium. Excessive ingestion of salt will accelerate the development of or aggravate vascular complications of diabetes. Diabetics with hypertension should be more cautious.

6. Abstention from smoking

As is well known, smoking is very harmful to health, and more so for diabetics because tobacco contains nicotine which stimulates the secretion of adrenalin to bring about a higher than normal concentration of sugar in blood, and thus has direct harm to diabetes. Heavy smoking can also reduce the volume of blood flow in coronary artery to speed up the progress of coronary heart disease. Nicotine can render the heart beat faster and blood pressure higher. A large amount of nicotine can inhibit and benumb the nerves. Diabetics, therefore, should not smoke and those who smoke must be determined to abstain from it.

7. Limited intake of food which increases blood sugar and blood lipid

A diabetic patient should not have food which can increase blood sugar like refined sugar, candies, pastry, chocolates, candied fruit, soda water, ice-cream, jam and toffee. Such food can be absorbed into the blood soon after being taken orally to cause the concentration of sugar in blood to rise rapidly and burden the islet β-cells.

Food which can increase the blood lipid, e. g. suet, lard, butter, cream, fat meat, chicken skin and cholesterol-rich food like the brain of livestock and yolk, should not be taken excessively, for they tend to give rise to diabetes complicated by cardiovascular troubles.

8. No drinking

The alcohol in wine or other alcoholic drinks contains no nutrient except providing thermal energy. The alcohol is mainly decomposed in the liver. Unfortunately, in diabetics, owing to the disturbance of glycometabolism, the glucose reserve in the liver is inadequate and the alcohol decomposing capacitiy of the liver is also poor. For these reasons, excessive drinking over a long period of time is likely to cause damage to the liver and lead to the rise of triglyceride in blood serum. A few patients under treatment of sulfaurea drugs tend to develop such symptoms as palpitation and shortness of breath after drinking. If a patient receiving injections of insulin drinks on an empty stomach, he is apt to develop hypoglycemia. The incidence of angiosclerosis and hypertension in diabetics is high and drinking over a long period of time will accelerate their development and progress. Although beer and rice wine contains only little alcohol, they should not be had to excess, and if they are drunk, their thermal energy should be calculated out and deducted from the staple food. Furthermore, it is not wise to drink on an empty stomach.

9. Do not eat much fruit

Although fruits contain nutrients most beneficial to health, they contain glucose too. Their blood sugar index (which reflects the concentration of blood sugar after eating) is rather high and they should, therefore, not be eaten in excess. A diabetic patient can select and include in his diet those fruits which contain less sugar and are suitable to his own condition. However, when his condition is not stable, they should also be shunned. When his condition is under good control and sugar concentration in both urine and blood is not high, he is justified in eating fruits in small quantity, say, 1-2 apples a day. If he prefers to have more fruit than he can afford, then he should take less staple food. For instance, every 200-250g of apple eaten is equal to 25g of staple food, which should be deducted accordingly. It is preferable for fruits to be eaten between meals when the blood sugar level is low.

The sugar content of different kinds of fruit varies. Reference can be found in the following table.

Tab. 3-5 Nutritional Values of Common Fruits (per 100g)

Fruits	Protein (g)	Fat (g)	Sugar (g)	Quantity of heat (joules)
Water melon	0.6	0.4	5.0	108.9
Hami muskmelon	0.4	0.3	8.8	167.6
Grape	0.4	0.3	8.2	167.6
Grapefruit	0.7	0.6	12.2	238.8
Orange	0.6	0.1	12.2	217.9
Tangerine	0.7	0.1	10.0	184.4
Apple	0.4	0.5	13.0	243.0
Pear	0.1	0.1	9.0	155.0
Peach	0.8	0.01	10.0	171.8
Apricot	1.2	0.0	11.1	205.3
Strawberry	1.0	0.6	5.7	134.0
Cherry	1.2	0.3	7.9	163.4
Persimmon	0.7	0.1	10.8	171.8
Pomegranate	1.5	1.6	16.8	368.7
Chinese date	1.2	0.2	23.2	414.8
Lychee	0.7	0.6	13.3	255.6
Fresh longan	1.2	0.1	16.2	297.0
Banana	1.2	0.6	19.5	368.7
Pineapple	0.6	0.2	12.2	221.0
Sugarcane	0.2	0.5	12.4	230.0

Foods Often Used to Treat Diabetes

1. Chinese yam

It can be used alone as food, or 250g of it is simmered in water every day to get a decoction as a substitute for tea, used on a long-term basis; or 100g of it is stewed together with a pork's pancreas

and both the broth and yam are to be taken.
2. Ricefield eel
Every day 60-90g of the fish meat is cut into shreds or pieces and cooked for a dish for a Type II diabetic patient.
3. Balsam pear
50-100g of fresh balsam pear is cooked for a dish for one meal, 2-3 times a day; or it is made into a dried powder, 7-12g of which is swallowed with lukewarm water, 3 times a day.
4. Pumpkin
500g of pumpkin is boiled and eaten up in a day; or 10g of its powder is taken, 2 times a day, for a long period of time. It is most effective for a patient whose fasting blood sugar value is about 8.4mml/L.
5. Taro
It is boiled for food, 60-90g a time, 2 times a day. It should not be eaten or should be eaten in small amount for those with abdominal distention.
6. Duck meat
One old duck is slaughtered, skinned, eviscerated and washed clean. Then 100g of gordon seed is inserted into the duck, which is stewed together in an earthen pot with proper amount of water on a slow fire for about 2 hours. Put in proper amount of salt before eating.
7. Pork pancreas
A pork's pancreas and 60g of Chinese yam are stewed together, then put in proper amount of salt, drink the broth and eat the pancreas and yam. Or a pork's pancreas and 50g of corn floss are stewed together in water for a decoction daily, 10 days as a course of treatment. Or a pork's pancreas is washed clean, baked dry and ground into a powder, which is taken with lukewarm water, 3-6g a time, 3 times a day.
8. Celery
It is washed clean and mashed to get the juice for oral use, 3-4 tablespoonfuls a time, 3 times a day, for 7 days on end.

9. Spinach

200-400g of spinach is washed clean and chopped, 10-20g of membrane of chicken's gizzard is baked dry and ground into a powder. The two things are simmered in a pot for a decoction to drink, 2-3 doses a day.

10. Wax gourd

1 000g of it is boiled in a small amount of water, then it is wrung in a piece of clean cloth to get the juice as a drink, 2 times a day.

11. Onion

100g of onion is soaked in boiling water and then cut into thin shreds, which is mixed with proper amount of soy sauce as a dish to go with staple food, 2 times a day.

12. Mung bean

It is boiled in water for a juice or cooked with rice for a porridge.

13. Soybean

It has some effect in the prevention and treatment of diabetes if it is eaten frequently.

14. Mushroom

It has some elements which can lower the level of blood sugar and blood-lipid. It can be cooked for a dish.

15. Bean curd

It contains rich high quality vegetable protein but very little sugar and so it is most suitable for diabetics as food.

16. Glutinous rice

30g of popped glutinous rice together with 30g of mulberry bark is boiled in water for an oral decoction, 2 times a day.

17. Millet

It can be cooked for a porridge or ground into flour to make pancake, etc.

18. Sorghum

The sorghum grains can be cooked for porridge or its flour is mixed with that of millet to make pancake.

19. Guava

Drink 1-3 galsses of its juice after a meal or 50g of dried guava and one balsam pear are decocted in water for a drink, 1-2 times a day.

20. Carrot

In modern medical research, an element which can lower the concentration of sugar in blood is extracted from dried carrot. Fresh carrot juice has hypoglycemic action. Carrot can be eaten in various ways—raw, as a juice or mash.

21. Asparagus

It can be boiled, stir-fried or just sliced and mixed with dressings.

22. Spinach

It can be cooked for a cold dish, stir-fried for a dish or cooked for a soup. Spinach soup with the inside membrane of chicken gizzard which is baked and powered has an auxilliary curative effect on diabetes.

23. Water spinach

Scalded in boiling water, it is mixed with dressings for a dish; or it is stir-fried with or without meat for a dish. 60g of fresh water spinach stalk and 30g of corn floss can be boiled for an oral decoction.

24. Water melon

It is eaten fresh but not too much. 15g of both water melon rind and wax gourd rind and 12g of snakegourd root can be boiled for a decoction to be drunk like tea.

25. Leek

150-250g of leek can be eaten every day, stir-fried or cooked in a thick soup without salt. But it should not be used after the Chinese solar term Pure Brightness (beginning on April 4, 5 or 6).

26. Pear

It is eaten raw or pounded to get its juice, or its juice is simmered and thickened as a paste for oral use.

27. Pomelo, orange and tangerine

They contain insulin-like composition and can be eaten raw.

28. White hycinth bean
The bean is uncoated and ground into flour, which is mixed with the decoction of snakegourd root and honey to prepare pills as big as a Chinese parasol seed. The pills are coated with gold foil. 20 - 30 pills a day taken in 2 times with a decoction of snakegourd root.

29. Cowpea
100-150g of cowpea with pods is decocted in water for an oral dose. Husked bean can be cooked with rice for porridge.

30. Pea
It can be boiled for a soup or stir-fried for a dish but should not be eaten too much at a time. Both the pea and pea seedling can be eaten simply after boiling or can be pressed for juice to drink.

Simple Food Recipes Commonly Used for Diabetes

1. Soybean buns
Ingredients:

Soybean flour	200g
Corn flour	200g
Wheat flour	100g
Fresh yeast	proper amount

The three kinds of flour are mixed with the yeast already dissolved in a proper amount of lukewarm water (30℃) to make dough. When the dough is well kneaded, it is let alone for fermentation. When fully fermented, the dough is kneaded and made into buns, which are then cooked with steam. The steamed soybean buns are a very satisfactory staple food for diabetics.

2. Stir-fried onion with slices of pork pancreas
Ingredients:

Onion	150g
Pork pancreas	2 whole pieces
Rice wine	
Ginger	

Oil	
Salt	
Gourmet powder	all in proper amount

After being scalded in boiling water, the pancreas is cut into slices, which are then cured with rice wine, ginger juice and salt for 15 minutes. The onion is cut into thin shreds and is stir-fried in hot oil. Then add in pancreas slices, heat to boil and add salt and gourmet powder to proper taste.

3. Stewed pork with dried cowpea and dried bean curd
Ingredients:

Dried cowpea	100g
Dried bean curd	100g
Lean pork	250g
Cooking wine	
Soy sauce	
Gourmet powder	all in proer amount

Soak the dried cowpea in boiling water until it is soft. Let water drip off and then cut the cowpea into pieces. Cut the dried bean curd into small cubes, and meat into small pieces. Simmer everything together with spices on a slow fire till overdone.

4. Wax gourd slices with green onion and sesame oil
Ingredients:

Wax gourd	500g
Green onion	50g
Sesame oil	
Salt	
Gourmet powder	all in proper amount

Slice the gourd and then decoct it with the rind in water for 10 minutes. Take out the gourd slices, cut off the rind and leave the decoction as a drink. Stir-fry green onion in hot sesame oil, add in salt and gourmet powder and then mix everything for a dish.

5. Slices of bamboo shoot and pork tripe
Ingredients:

Pork tripe	250g
Bamboo shoot	100g

Garlic	1 clove
Rice wine	
Salt	
Gourmet powder	
Cooking oil	all in proper amount

Wash the tripe clean, cut it to thin slices which are scalded by pouring boiling water on them. Cut the bamboo shoot also into slices, which are scalded in boiling water. Cut the garlic into grains. Heat the oil in the pan, put in garlic grains and stir-fry till it gives off a good smell. Add in tripe slices and rice wine to stir-fry, then add in bamboo shoot slices and salt, heat to boil and add in gourmet powder before serving.

6. Stewed pork pancreas and Chinese yam
Ingredients:

Pork pancreas	1 whole piece
Chinese yam	60g

Stew the two in water and add in salt to proper taste. Eat 1-2 times a day.

7. Stewed pork pancreas with sea slug and egg
Ingredients:

Pork pancreas	1 whole piece
Sea slug	1 piece
Egg	1
Oil	
Soy sauce	proper amount

First soak the dry sea slug soft and then slice it. Stew the pancreas and sea slug together till thoroughly done. Add in the shelled boiled egg and some soy sauce. One dish a day.

8. Porridge of astragalus and Chinese yam
Ingredients:

Astragalus root	30g
Chinese yam	60g

Yam is ground into a flour. Astragalus is simmered in water to get 300ml of decoction, which is filtered and added into yam flour to cook a porridge. 1-2 times a day.

9. Stewed rabbit with wolfberry fruit
Ingredients:
Wolfberry fruit	15g
Rabbit meat	250g

Stew the ingredients in proper amount of water till they are thoroughly done. Add in salt, eat the meat and drink the broth, once a day.

10. Porridge of Chinese yam and coix seed
Ingredients:
Chinese yam	60g
Coix seed	30g

Boil them together for a porridge, 2 times a day.

11. Porridge of pork pancreas and coix seed
Boil a pork's pancreas in water. Take it out, add 60g of coix seed into the broth to cook a porridge. The boiled pancreas is served with salt to go with staple food.

12. Stewed pork pancreas and astragalus root
Ingredients:
Pork pancreas	1 whole piece
Astragalus root	30g
Salt	proper amount

The pancreas and the astragalus root are stewed together till thoroughly done. Then add in proper amount of salt. Eat the pancreas and drink the broth.

13. Stewed crucian carp with tea
Ingredients:
Live crucian carp	500g
Green tea leaves	10g

A live crucian carp weighing about 500g is killed, eviscerated and scaled. Stuff the green tea leaves into it, put it on a plate and steam it. No salt should be used. One fish a day.

14. Porridge with Chinese yam and longan
Ingredients:
Chinese yam	30g
Longan	15g

Lychee	10g
Schisandra fruit	10g
Rice	150g

Cook all the ingredients together into a porridge in the usual way.

15. Ricefield eel
Eat plenty of ricefield eel because it contains hypoglycemic composition and is very good to diabetic patients.

16. Soup of pork pancreas and corn floss
Ingredients:

Pork pancreas	200g
Corn floss	30g

Decoct the two in water for a decoction taken in 2 times a day.

17. Soup of pork, corn floss and snakegourd root
Ingredients:

Corn floss	90g
Snakegourd root	30g
Lean pork	100g

First stew the pork, and when it is about done, add in corn floss and snakegourd root. Boil on on a slow fire for a medicated broth. Drink the broth and eat the meat.

18. Stir-fried vegetable shreds
Ingredients:

Celery	450g
Carrot	80g
Dried mushroom	50g (soaked with water)
Vegetable oil	50g
Salt	2g
Chopped green onion	5g
Gourmet powder	1g

All the ingredients are cooked in the usual way that a stir-fried dish is done.

19. Soup of clam and balsam pear
Ingredients:

Balsam pear	250g

Clam meat	100g
Oil and salt	proper amount

Boil balsam pear and clam meat together for a soup, and add in oil and salt to proper taste.

Kinesitherapy for Diabetes

A Brief Introduction of Kinesitherapy for Diabetes

Kinesitherapy refers to physical exercise used to prevent and treat diseases. This therapy, dietotherapy and pharmacotherapy are collectively known as the three principal therapies for diabetes.

China is the first country in the world to propose and practice treating diabetes with kinesitherapy. Early in the Sui Dynasty 1 300 years ago, the famous physician Chao Yuanfang realized the significance of kinesitherapy. He proposed in *General Treatise on Causes and Symptoms of Diseases* that diabetics "should walk for 120 steps or as many as a thousand steps prior to meals." The famous physician of Tang Dynasty, Wang Tao, proposed that diabetic patients should "have a walk right after meals and should not sit down until they feel comfortable in the abdomen." He also pointed out: "One should not lie down right after eating one's fill and sit all day long. A man should do some work but should not work too long and to exhaustion. Moreover, one should not do what one cannot." Many physicians of every generation after them have made brilliant expositions on the importance of kinesitherapy in the treatment of diabetes.

Professor Staikmann, the director of German Research Institute of Athletic Physiology, once said: "Proper amount of physical exercise is the best way of prevention and treatment of 'civilization diseases' and is a most ideal form of human health activities." In another word, different kinds of physical exercise in combination with proper diet planning and a proper balance between work and rest are important measures to prevent and treat "civilization diseases" (diabetes, obesity, hypertension, coronary heart disease, arteriosclerosis, etc.).

Clinically, a large number of examples have demonstrated the important role that kinesitherapy has played in the prevention and treatment of diabetes. It has been proved that in some mild non-insulin-dependent cases, the diabetes can well be brought under control by only kinesitherapy in combination with diet control.

The Beneficial Effects of Physical Exercise on Diabetics

1. The effect on carbohydrate metabolism

Experiments have been made that after 30 minutes of physical exercise, the blood sugar can reduce 0.67-0.89mmol/L, the consumption of insulin is decreased, and the overburden of islet cells is reduced. Those who are engaged in regular physical exercise can improve their carbohydrate metabolism over a long period of time. This is because physical exercise of each time improves the sensitivity of glucose to insulin. It can be inferred from this that if one wants to improve his carbohydrate metabolism on a long-term basis, he must persist in long-term regular exercise, i.e. he has to do physical exercise in 3-5 days of a week. It is believed after a great deal of research that physical exercise has extraordinary effect on patients whose glucose tolerance is abnormal, or who suffer from mild-moderate diabetes, or whose fasting blood sugar value is less than 11.1mmol/L because physical exercise can stimulate the metabolism of carbohydrate and reduce the burden of islets.

During physical activity, the thermal energy that the body requires comes mainly from muscle glycogen and hepatic glycogen, the utilization of which needs the promotion of insulin. When the muscles contract during physical activity, carrier protein for glucose transportation is produced around the muscular cells to promote the glucose decomposition, and to increase anaerobic glycolysis and utilization of glucose when the muscular cells are in absence of oxygen, and as a result, blood sugar content is lowered. Physical activities, therefore, can promote glucose metabolism to lower the blood sugar.

2. The effect on fat metabolism

Most of the fats in the human body are triglyceride and cholesterol, which, together with apolipoprotein and phospholipid and in various proportions, compose lipoprotein-cholesterol-triglyceride complexes, that is, low density lipoprotein, cholesterol, very low density lipoprotein cholesterol and high density lipoprotein cholesterol. The higher the concentration of low density lipoprotein cholesterol in the blood, the greater the possibility of arteriosclerosis, and the more likely the diabetic will suffer from complications of disorder of the great vessels. Elevated concentration of high density lipoprotein cholesterol in the blood can prevent the arteries from sclerosis while its lowered concentration will accelerate development of arteriosclerosis. Regular long-term physical exercise will lower the concentration of low density lipoprotein cholesterol in blood and triglyceride in serum and increase the concentration of high density lipoprotein. All these changes help to prevent diabetes and treat its complications of great vessels. Moreover, diabetics invariably suffer from a disturbance of lipo-metabolism and kinesitherapy is also beneficial to the regulation of blood-lipid.

3. The effect on cardiovascular vessels

Coronary heart disease is one of the principal complications and a leading cause of death in patients of type II diabetes. Statistics of an epidemiological survey show that the incidence of coronary heart disease evidently decreases in people who manage to do regular long-term physical exercise. This suggests that physical exercise is beneficial to the cardiovascular system, for exercise can regulate blood-lipid, lower blood pressure, increase the contractive power of cardiac muscles and heart volume at end-diastolic phase, decrease the response of sympathetic nervous system to stress, and minimize the possibility of attacks of angina pectoris.

4. The effect on body weight

Obesity is the principal cause of insulin-resistance in type II diabetics, for which reason, reducing body weight is a most important means to improve the control of blood sugar for type II diabetes. Energy is consumed during physical exercise, which will help the oxidation of fat and reduce fat in an all-round way from the body. Long-term and persistent physical exercise will make a person more muscular. Since muscles are the chief locations where glucose is converted into glycogen, stronger muscles can store more glycogen and increase the sensitivity of insulin, which is beneficial to the control of diabetes.

5. The effect on skeletal and muscular systems

With increase of age and decrease of exercise, a diabetic patient tends to develop osteoporosis and incurs ostealgia, bone fracture and deformity. On the contrary, physical exercise makes the skeleton broader and the content of minerals in the bones richer. The metabolism in bones is more active in people who often do physical exercise than in ordinary people. When the burden the skeleton bears is increased, the bone density is also increased and content of minerals in the bone is higher. In addition, physical exercise produces a remarkable action on the concentration of insulin in plasma and the uptaking and utilizing of blood sugar by skeletal muscles. During exercise, the secretion of insulin is inhibited so the concentration of insulin in plasma is low. However, when the skeletal muscles are in contractive movements, the uptaking of blood sugar by their cells are distinctively increased. It is generally believed that during physical exercise, the blood inside the body is redistributed. The blood flow to the internal organs decreases, the capillaries of the muscles in motion are dilated, and a large quantity of insulin-rich blood flows into the muscles in motion. On the other hand, the potency of insulin becomes greater due to the changes in affinity between receptors and insulin. In the recovery phase after physical exercise, the sensitivity of skeletal muscles to insulin increases and can last for as long as 4 hours. It is not difficult to understand from the above evidences that physical exercise increases the synthesis of muscle glycogen, improves muscle metabolism, increases myodynamia and muscular mobility.

6. The effect on other aspects

It has been found in research that physical exercise can increase the blood volume in circulation and oxygen-carrying capacity of erythrocytes, improve the fiber dissolution and prevent thrombosis. Physical exercise can also relieve one of his mental stress, anxiety and depression, and improve his psychic reaction and the function of immunological system and can thus build up his health, better his psychology and improve the quality of his life.

Adverse Effect of Improper Physical Exercise on Diabetics

Although physical exercise has so many advantages mentioned above and even more advantages that have not been understood, yet improper physical exercise cannot build up health and bring diabetes under control but may give rise to many adverse effects, do harm to health and even endanger the patient's life. Therefore, it is no good to advocate physical exercise blindly. Improper physical exercise may produce harmful effects on the following types of diabetics.

1. Diabetics with serious cardiovascular complications

(1) In cases with coronary heart disease, exercise may cause arrhythmia and cardiac functional insufficiency.

(2) During physical exercise, the blood pressure may be overly elevated, and therefore, patients with severe hypertension should

not do physical exercise.

(3) In patients with postural hypotension, the blood pressure may drop drastically due to sudden change of posture as the exercise comes to a sudden stop.

2. Diabetics with pathologic changes in micrangia

(1) In patients with angioma of the micrangia or proliferative lesion in the optical fundus, strenuous exercise may cause fluctuation of blood pressure and increase blood pressure, often leading to hemorrhage as the result of rupture of angioma or frail neoformative vessels.

(2) In cases of diabetic renopathy, decreased renal blood supply may result after exercise to aggravate renal ischemia so that proteinuria may occur and the content of blood urea nitrogen will be increased.

(3) Exercise may accelerate the damage of micrangia.

3. Diabetics with metabolic disturbance

Patients who are using insulin or sulfaurea drugs may be attacked by hypoglycemia to develop hypoglycemic coma during or after exercise. In the cases of severe deficiency of insulin, physical exercise does not lower the blood sugar but increases it or even gives rise to ketoacidosis.

In addtion, physical exercise may bring about unfavourable effects on patients who suffer from acute infection, hepatic or renal failure, heart failure, severe arrhythmia, acute myocarditis and pulmonary heart disease.

The Indications of Kinesitherapy

Type II (non-insulin-dependent) diabetics, especially obese patients, are encouraged to take up kinesitherapy. Kinesitherapy is also suitable for Type I (insulin-dependent) patients whose condition has been improved or is under control after having been treated with other therapies, and for diabetic patients who are treated with oral hypoglycemic agents or injection of small dosage of insulin.

Diabetic patients with hyperlipemia, arteriosclerosis, peripheral neuritis, mild hypertension or coronary heart disease can take up kinesitherapy but should not do strenuous or heavy load exercise lest the complications should be aggravated.

Contraindications to Kinesitherapy

1. Diabetes complicated by severe trouble of the heart, brain, kidney or retina, acute infections, and during pregnancy.
2. Type I diabetes not under good control.
3. Patients who cannot control their diet.
4. Patients who are fasting and those who are suffering from diarrhea, vomiting or those who have hypoglycemic potential.

Points for Attention During Kinesitherapy

If a diabetic patient is to set about doing physical exercise, he should begin with light and short-timed exercise, proceed in an orderly way and step by step, keep on exercise perseveringly and take a proper amount of exercise. The exercise should vary with an individual patient's own condition and circumstances.

1. The intensity and duration of exercise should depend on a patient's actual condition. In principle, it is better to practice exercises which are not strenuous and are easy to keep up.
2. A patient should do physical exercise perseveringly and should not stop it unless an acute complication occurs.
3. Since exercise can lower blood sugar, patients who are under treatment with medicines or insulin are likely to have hypoglycemia. In order to prevent the occurrence of hypoglycemia during or after exercise, it is better to take exercise 2 hours after meal. The patient should bring candy or biscuits along with him so that he can eat some in case he has the feeling of hypoglycemia.
4. Patients who are under insulin treatment should not do physical exercise at the time that insulin is in full action. For example, if one is given insulin in the early morning, special care

should be taken to prevent hypoglycemia when he does exercise at 10-11 a.m.

5. Insulin-dependent patients must be careful not to do exercises in the early morning before the injection of insulin, for the level of insulin in blood is so low then that ketosis is very likely to be induced.

6. In patients with pathological changes in the ocular fundus, the rise of blood pressure and acceleration of blood flow after exercise may give rise to or aggravate hemorrhage in the ocular fundus.

7. In patients with diabetic renopathy, blood supply for the kidneys is reduced after exercise, which may cause exacerbation of renal ischemia, increase of protein in urine and high content of urea nitrogen in blood.

8. Diabetics with arteriosclerosis should also take physical exercise cautiously because arteriosclerosis is often accompanied by coronary heart disease and exercise may lead to myocardial ischemia and arrhythmia or even painless myocardial infarction.

9. When a diabetic patient is affected with acute gastroenteritis or pneumonia, exercise should be brought to a pause immediately.

10. In case of serious pathological changes of the peripheral nerves and blood vessels, exercise may promote the development of ulcers in feet, and therefore the feet should be checked each time after exercise.

11. Comfortable shoes and socks of proper size should be worn and other protective equipment should be used.

12. Before kinesitherapy, a patient must go to a hospital to have a complete physical examination.

13. Kinesitherapy must go parallel with dietotherapy.

Contents and Methods of Kinesitherapy

A patient should decide on, in light of his own age and physical condition, exercise forms which he is fond of and which are suitable to him. It is preferable to take outdoor exercise such as callisthenics, fast walking, jogging, swimming, shadow boxing, shadow boxing with sword, disco dance for the aged, etc.

1. Callisthenics

(1) Alternate fast and slow walking. Walk fast and slow alternately in fresh air with big strides for 10-15 minutes each time.

(2) Arm-propping exercise. Stand upright facing a wall at an arm's length with both hands against the wall to practise arm-propping exercise by bending and stretching the arms alternately (The movements are the same as in push-up). Exhale while bending the arms and inhale while stretching them. Practice for 20-30 times in each session. The exercise can strengthen the muscles in the upper limbs.

(3) Squatting exercise. Start from standing upright with the feet apart as wide as the shoulders, then squat (halfway or completely) and stand up alternately. Exhale while squatting down and inhale on standing up, 20-30 times as a session. The exercise helps to strengthen the muscles of the lower limbs.

(4) Bending-extending spine exercise. Stand upright in front of a wall at an arm's length with the back facing the wall. Bend the body forward with the arms stretching straight, try hard to reach the ground with the finger-tips and exhale deeply at the same time. Then stand up, extend the body backward with the arms stretching straight to reach the wall and inhale slowly at the same time. Repeat the movements 10-20 times in each session. The exercise can strengthen the muscles of the back and abdomen.

(5) Arm-stretching with deep breath. Stand upright, raise the arms, spread them out and meanwhile inhale deeply. Then exhale completely on lowering the arms to the original posture. Repeat the exercise 8-10 times. The exercise is good for strengthening diaphragmatic muscles and respiratory muscles. It is also beneficial to the removal of stagnant blood in the liver and to the recovery from muscular fatigue.

The exercises described above can be done in the early morning or both morning and evening.

2. Walking

Walk at the speed of 5-7 kilometers per hour for 30 minutes a time. This exercise is suitable for type II and obese diabetics for it can strengthen the heart muscles and reduce body weight. During walking the fastest heart rate should be controlled under 120 beats per minute and the body should be upright with the head up, the eyes looking straight ahead, the arms swinging naturally and breathing smoothly.

Walk at the speed of 60-80 paces a minute for 30 minutes. This exercise is suitable for diabetic patients with a rather serious condition and old age or type I patients with a mild condition.

3. Jogging

By jogging, it is meant to run at a slow speed for a long distance. During jogging, the muscles contract rhythmatically. This contraction depends on energy generated from oxidation of the nutritional substances in the body—mainly sugar and fats. Jogging, therefore, can regulate the metabolism in the body, including sugar and fats, and has a definite effect in the prevention and treatment of diabetes, obesity and hyperlipemia. Besides, jogging has good effects on nervous system, motor system and hematopoietic system, and is thus of great benefit in preventing some complications of diabetes. However, care should be taken that the patient practicing jogging should be well looked after medically to prevent accidents.

4. Swimming

Swimming at normal speed consumes about 21-84kJ of energy every minute, and in winter more energy is used. If one remains in water of 12℃ for 4 minutes, the heat energy radiated is equal to that used in one hour on land, so swimming can promote the consumption of surplus fat in the body and it is the most suitable exercise for obese diabetics.

5. Taiji Quan (Shadow boxing)

A traditional health-building exercise in China, shadow boxing has included the essence of all ancient Chinese callisthenics in one. It is characterized by leisurely, natural, graceful, and supple movements. Training both internal and external Qigong, it makes the respiration, thoughts and movements harmoniously united in the exercise. The movements of the boxing are gentle and slow but continuous without stopping just like flowing water. The exercise intensity can be regulated at the patient's will. It is one of the best health preserving exercises. It has been proved in practice that shadow boxing is a good method for treating chronic maladies, a miraculous cure for the aged to preserve health and prolong life. As far as diabetics are concerned, it is capable of regulating metabolism, blood sugar, blood-lipid and blood pressure, and has been proved to have definite effect in the prevention and treatment of diabetes, especially diabetes due to obesity or complicated by troubles of the heart, blood vessels and peripheral nerves.

6. Five Mimic-animal Boxing

This is an ancient physical exercise method in China, whose designer is the famous ancient Chinese doctor Hua Tuo of the Han Dynasty. Having summerized all the experience before him in mimicking the movements of birds and animals, including the movements of tiger, deer, bear, ape and birds, to build up health, he designed a set of setting-up exercises. Regular practice of this boxing is helpful in nourishing the brain, improving eyesight and cardiac and pulmonary functions, strengthening the kidney and the waist, preventing and relieving rigidity of joints, and consolidating body constitution.

7. Eight-section Callisthenics

This is a set of Chinese folk setting-up exercises consisting of eight parts. It is very easy to learn and perform and has an evident body-building effect. Its movements are very natural, graceful, gentle and supple, with every action looking like a graceful model. By stretching, extending and bending the body and limbs and relaxing and contracting muscles, the exercises can promote the flow of Qi in the channels and collaterals and circulation of Qi and blood in the viscera to strengthen the body resistance, prevent diseases and prolong life. As all the movements in the exercises are gentle and slow and the exercise are not strenuous, they are most suitable for middle-aged and aged diabetics, especially the weak ones.

8. Others

A diabetic patient can select, according to his or her own condition and interest, one to two from such sports as shadow boxing with sword, badminton, table tennis, croquet, billiards and disco dance for the middle-aged and aged, to practice regularly. In combination with dietotherpay, these physical exercises help the patient to bring the blood sugar under satisfactory control and reduce the incidence of complications.

Qigong Therapy for Diabetes

A Brief Account of Qigong Therapy

1. A brief account of Qigong

Qigong is one of the gems of China's cultural heritage and a magnificent bright pearl in the treasure-house of TCM. It is the summerization of experience in consciousness-guided self-control and self-regulation of life activities gained in the course of Chinese people's long struggle against nature and diseases, and is a unique self-training exercise for both the body and the mind. Qigong regulates the physiological condition of the body by exercising the mind, respiration and postures, and is, therefore, of great importance in building up health, developing wisdom, preventing and curing diseases and prolonging life. In recent years, great attention has been paid to this ancient science by modern people. A great upsurge of Qigong occurred in a worldwide range, and Qigong has played a more and more important role in the prevention and treatment of diseases.

The development of Qigong is a long story. *Lu's Spring and Autumn Annals* recorded that in the legendary dynasty called Tang founded by Emperor Yao more than 4 000 years ago, "For those whose muscles and bones cowered and stiffened so that they could not move properly due to obstruction and stagnation of Qi in the body, dances were designed to remove the stagnation and obstruction." The Spring and Autumn and Warring States are the time periods in which Qigong came into being. *Jade Pendant Inscription on Qigong* is a complete work on Qigong written at the time. In "On Acupuncture Therapy", a chapter in *Plain Questions*, the following was written: "To treat chronic renal diseases, one can face the south at *yin* time period (3-5 a.m.), relax his mind, clear the mind of stray thoughts, hold his breath seven times, each time craning the neck slightly to send the breath down as if a very hard object were being swallowed. Repeat seven times to cause the tongue to produce saliva, and the more, the better." It can be seen from these description that special medical Qigong was developed to treat diseases at the time. *Notes to the Book of Changes Left from the Zhou Dynasty* written in the Qin or Han Dynasty is a classical work on Qigong for the pellet-school of Taoism. During the Wei Dynasty, Jin Dynasty and Southern and Northern State Periods, Qigong grew more sophiscated. The prosperity of Buddhism and development of Taoism also accelerated the development of Qigong. Sui Dynasty and Tang Dynasty were the prosperous period of Qigong. Special Qigong exercises for diabetes evolved then. *General Treatise on Etiology and Symptoms of Diseases*, written by Chao Yuanfang during the Sui Dynasty, recorded a Qigong method for treating diabetes called "Qigong therapy for diabetes by removing stagnation and obstruction". This is suitable for diabetes involving the upper Jiao and marked chiefly by thirst, polydipsia and dysuria. The Song Dynasty, Jin Dynasty and Yuan Dynasty were periods of popularization and improvement of Qigong. In the Ming and Qing dynasties, there was new progress in the systematization and summerization of the literature of Qigong. For example, *Eight Works on Life Preservation* by Gao Lian of the Ming Dynasty is a monograph on health preservation through Qigong exercise. In *Records of Traditional Chinese and Western Medicine in Combination* written by Zhang Xichun in the late Qing Dynasty, there is a sound analysis of clearing the obstruction in the Ren and Du Channels by an active endogenous substance gained through

Qigong practice. After the founding of the People's Republic of China, Qigong made rapid progress. In 1953, Liu Guizhen and others set out to establish a Qigong sanatorium in the city of Tangshan, and conducted treatment of diseases with Qigong. Good therapeutic effects were achieved in the treatment of gastrointestinal diseases and diabetes by a combination of the patient's own Qigong exercise and treatment with Qi emitted by doctors. Valuable experience was gained, which was a great contribution to the later development and popularization of Qigong.

Qigong refers to the way of the training of Qi, cultivation of Qi and application of Qi. It is also known as "life preservation exercise", "health conservation exercise", "expiration and inspiration exercise", "physical and breathing exercise", and "mind concentration exercise". "Qi" refers to the genuine Qi in traditional Chinese Medicine, or known as internal Qi. *Miraculous Pivot* defined it as this: "The so-called genuine Qi is an integrated substance of the congenital Qi inherited and the acquired Qi derived from food and air that fill up the body." It is held in TCM that the genuine Qi is the basic substance and motivating force for the life activities of the human body. It consists of the inborn Qi (i. e. primordial Qi or congenital Qi), which is inherited from one's parents, and the acquired Qi, which is air breathed and essence obtained from the food eaten. The Qi obtained from Qigong exercise or training refers to the Qi derived from the primordial Qi, pectoral Qi, nutrative Qi and defensive Qi which are trained through the three regulation methods and have developed special functions and gained more energy. This Qi can congregate and diffuse under the control of the mind, and can exchange with the outside world. It is referred to as "internal Qi" or "external Qi" of Qigong. Therefore, the so-called "training or exercise of Qi" frequently referred to in Qigong practice refers to the training of genuine Qi.

Since 1978, the Shanghai Traditional Chinese Medicine Research Institute has cooperated with the institutions concerned in the detection study of the material basis of the external Qi produced by Qigong by means of modern scientific instruments, and has proved that the external Qi emitted by some Qigong masters can produce a series of physical effects. Also, in the external Qi, infrared rays, electrostatic charges, magnetic fields, particle beams, etc. have been detected with modern scientific instruments. It has also been proved in animal experiments that external Qi has many physiological effects. All these have proved that Qigong is not disembodied but an energy substance with many motional forms. The evidence has provided a reliable scientific basis for the clinical application and popularization of Qigong.

Qi exhibits the following characteristics: ① Universality. It exists in everyone and everything. ② Systematization. Not only the heavenly Qi and earthly Qi are interlinked, but there is a Qi system within the human body—a small "heaven and earth". ③ Dissemination. Qi has the property of ductility, diffusion, proliferation and mobility. ④ Excitation. The external Qi acting on a patient can stimulate the Qi in the patient's body. ⑤ Synchronism. Qi of similar frequency and nature interact to produce resonance and excite things synchronically and rapidly. ⑥ Sensitivity. Everybody has varied sensitivity to Qi. ⑦ Controllability. The Qi in the body can be controlled by the mind.

Qigong has the following three prominent characteristics: ① Self-exercise of both the body and the mind; ② Arousing the self-regulating physiological function of the body, and ③ Bringing the body's latent potentialities into full play to produce a kind of psiphenomenal extraordinary power which is out of the ordinary physiological state.

2. Location, direction and time for Qigong exercise

Man and nature form an organic whole. A man is a small universe and is closely linked with the natural Qi. Usually, a quiet and peaceful place should be selected for Qigong exercises. When one conducts Qigong exercises outdoors, it is imperative to choose a good natural environment with fresh air, trees and flowers. It should be borne in mind never to practice Qigong in the vicinity of dead or dying trees and graveyards.

The chapter "On Regulation of Mental Activities in Accordance With the Changes of Four Seasons" in *Plain Questions* laid stress on the principle of "nourishing Yang in spring and summer and nourishing Yin in autumn and winter." The six two-hour periods of *zi*, *chou*, *yin*, *mao*, *chen* and *si* are six Yang periods while the six two-hour periods of *wu*, *wei*, *shen*, *you*, *xu* and *hai* are six Yin periods. Ancient Chinese people believed that during the six Yang periods, the external world was filled with living Qi while during the six Yin periods, with dead Qi, and so Qigong should be practiced in Yang periods to replenish Yang Qi, but should not be practiced or should be done less in Yin periods. However, those who are deficient of Yin can do more practice in the Yin periods to help retain abundant primordial Qi which will in turn benefit the storage and maintenance of Yang Qi. For diabetes arising from hyperactivity of fire due to Yin deficiency, the patient may do Qigong exercise more in the Yin periods. Beginners may practice Qigong mainly in the early morning and evening according to their own condition. Practitioners who have reached a certain level should usually choose the two-hour periods of *zi*, *wu*, *mao* and *you* to do Qigong exercises, concentrating on training Qi during *zi* and *wu* periods and on nourishing Qi during *mao* and *you* periods. As far as a particular individual is concerned, he should choose the right time to practice Qigong in view of his own constitution and condition of illness. For instance, *hai* and *zi* periods are good for regulating the kidney, *mao* and *yin* periods for the liver, *si* and *wu* periods for the heart, *shen* and *you* for the lung, and *zi* period for regulating the Gall-bladder Channel, *chou* for the Liver Channel, *yin* for the Lung Channel, *mao* for the Large Intestine Channel, *chen*, *shu*, *chou* and *wei* for the Spleen Channel.

As a rule, beginners can conduct Qigong training facing the east or south, or facing the direction of the sun in the daytime, and moon at night. There is a saying among Taoists: "When someone wants to know where I am doing Qigong exercises, he just needs to look in the direction of the moon." That is to say, the direction one faces during Qigong practice varies with different days in a month as well as different time periods in a day. To do Qigong exercises facing the east and south benefits Yang while facing the west and north benefits Yin. When a well-trained practitioner chooses a location, takes the proper posture and becomes tranquilized, he should carefully discern which among the four directions of east, west, south and north when he faces can enable him to generate the strongest sensation of Qi. The one that can do would be the best for him.

3. The basic requirements for Qigong practitioners

(1) Combination of activity with tranquility: Suitable practice methods for training both dynamic and static Qigong should be selected. To conduct static Qigong is to train Qi and accumulate Qi while to practice dynamic Qigong is to help Qi circulate more smoothly in the limbs, bones, and channels and collaterals. Dynamic and static Qigong exercises can complement each other. Furthermore, in the practice of Qigong, it is required to follow the principle of "seeking tranquility in activity" and "activity in tranquility."

(2) Relaxation, tranquilization and naturalness: By relaxation, it is meant that during Qigong training, both the body and the mind should be fully relaxed. By tranquilization, it is meant that during practice, the mood should be kept peaceful and stable.

(3) Unity of the mind and Qi: "The Mind" refers to the mental activity of the practitioner during Qigong practice; "Qi" refers to the air breathed in and some sensation during practice. By unity it is meant that the mind and Qi should be united organically as one. Undue emphasis on either leading the activity of Qi by the mind or the mind's passively following Qi should be avoided.

(4) Concurrence of training and nourishing Qi: Training or exercising Qi refers to the practice of Qigong under powerful control of consciousness while nourishing Qi refers to the peaceful, relaxed, comfortable and tranquil state as the result of Qigong training, in which there should not be much thought and respiration. The training of Qi and nourishment of Qi are often conducted al-

ternately. If attention is only paid to nourishing Qi without exercising it, not much attainment can be made, whereas exercising Qi without nourishing it, the vitality and Qi will be consumed. Only by concurrently exercising and nourishing Qi can the quality of Qigong practice be improved and life be prolonged.

(5) A step-by-step sequence and persistence: In Qigong practice, haste brings no success, so one should proceed in order from the most elementary method to the advanced in accordance with the objective law of Qigong. Furthermore, the practice must be kept on perseveringly for a long time. If one changes his mind the moment he hears of something different in Qigong practice, or he practices fast and loose, or does it conscientiously for one day and suspends it for ten days, he will never be successful.

4. The key elements of Qigong practice

Posture, respiration and the mind are the three key concerns in Qigong practice. They are also known as "regulation of the body", "regulation of breathing" and "regulation of the mind".

(1) Regulation of the body, also known as posture or body method: It is very important for those who practice static Qigong or Daoyin Qigong to master correct postures. The postures commonly taken in Qigong practice are sitting, lying, standing and walking.

① Sitting posture: Sitting posture is further divided into three types: plain sitting, cross-legged sitting and back-supported sitting. In plain sitting posture, the practitioner should sit upright on a wide flat square stool or chair with the feet placed parallel on the floor and separated as wide as the two shoulders. Knees should be flexed to a 90° angle with the thighs, and the hands should be placed on the thighs with the palms downward. The arms should be curved naturally. The head should be raised upright with the lower jaw slightly drawn in. The back and waist should be straightened up with the shoulders relaxed and the chest slightly drawn in. The mouth and eyes should be loosely closed with the tip of the tongue raised against the hard palate. In the cross-legged posture, the practitioner should sit stably on a bed with the legs crossed and the feet under the legs. Something should be placed under the buttocks to raise them a little. The trunk should lean slightly forward. The two hands should gently grip each other with the left on top, the thumb of the right hand pressing the root of the ring finger of the left hand. The thumb and the middle finger of the left hand should come together and be placed in front of the chest. The back-supported sitting posture is much the same as the plain sitting posture except that the back may lean against a chairback or a sofa and the feet stretched a little straighter.

② Lying posture: The practitioner may lie on his back on a bed with the face up and head natural. The pillow should be of a comfortable height. The mouth and eyes should be slightly closed, the limbs held naturally straight, and the hands on either side of the body or overlapping on the abdomen. The practitioner may also lie on his side on a bed (either on the left or right side but usually on the right) with the waist and head slightly bent forward to form an arc. The head should rest level on the pillow with the mouth and eyes slightly closed. The palm of the top hand should be placed on the hip, and the other hand on the pillow. The underneath shank should be naturally stretched straight while the top leg should be put on it with the hip and knee flexed.

③ Standing posture: Stand with the feet shoulder-width apart and the head upright, the small of the back straightened up, the chest bent slightly forward, knees relaxed, and the arms raised and slightly flexed. The fingers should be separated naturally and kept in front of the chest or lower abdomen as if holding a ball. The palms are to be together as Buddhists do, or the hands overlapped on the lower abdomen with the left hand under the right for men and vice versa for women.

(2) Regulation of breathing: This refers to the respiration modes adopted by practitioners during Qigong exercise. The breathing methods commonly employed are as follows:

① Natural respiration method: This refers to usual respiration but should be more gentle than usual. This is the basic method for respiration training and is the common respiration style. It is further divided into thoracic natural respiration, abdominal natural respiration and mixed natural respiration.

② Orthodromic abdominal respiration: During inspiration, relax the abdominal muscles intentionally so that the abdomen will bulge out naturally but during expiration contract the abdominal muslces intentionally. As a rule, if the mind concentrates on the navel, it is easy to perform this respiration.

③ Counter-abdominal respiration: During inspiration, intentionally and gradually contract the abdominal muscles to draw the abdomen in while during expiration, relax the abdominal muscles consciously so that the abdomen will gradually bulge out. Generally when the practitioner can use this respiration method freely, he can start practicing anus-raising exercise during the respiration, that is, the levator ani muscle together with the pudendum contracts on inspiration and the levator ani muscle relaxes on expiration. A well-trained practitioner usually adopts this method of respiration.

④ Reading-word respiration: One way to practice this respiration is to shape the mouth on expiration as if to read a certain word but do not actually pronounce it. Take the six-character breathing method for example. On expiration, the lips are rounded to different shapes as if to read the Chinese characters *chui*, *hu*, *xi*, *ke*, *xu* and *si* but without actually pronouncing them. Another way is to pronounce a word on expiration. For example, in the *hai*-shouting exercise, during expiration, the word *hai* is shouted out loudly.

⑤ Other respiration methods: There are more respiration methods such as nose breathing method, nose-inhaling but mouth-exhaling method and mouth breathing method. Generally, when static Qigong is practiced, nose breathing is adopted, which can enable the breath to be deep, long, even and gentle.

(3) Regulation of the mind: This is also known as "mind method". The exercise of the mind is the most important link in Qigong training. The common methods are as follows:

① Mind concentration on the relaxation of the body: To relax the body consciously, this is a basic requirement in Qigong training. From the very beginning of a Qigong training session, the whole body, from head to feet, should be completely relaxed. The ability to take a good posture consciously and relax the body completely is the manifestation of the right way in regulation of the mind.

② Mind concentration on a part or an acupoint of the body: The acupoints the mind commonly concentrates on are the upper, middle and lower Dantian. Diabetic patients should make their mind concentrate on the lower Dantian or middle Dantian, or the acupoint Yongquan, but generally not on acupoints in the head lest fire of deficiency type may flare up to aggravate the disease.

③ Mind concentration on respiration: During a Qigong practice session, the number of respirations is counted in the mind, or the mind simply goes in and out with respiration without counting the number of respirations.

④ Mind concentration on words: For example, during inspiration, read silently in the mind the word "*jing*" (silence) while on expiration read silently the word "*song*" (relaxation).

⑤ The most commonly used acupoint for mind concentration is Dantian: There is a Dantian point in the upper, middle and lower respectively. The upper Dantian is generally believed to be the acupoint Baihui, which is located in the center of the head top, or the acupoint Yintang, which is between the two eye-brows. The middle Dantian is at the acupoint Shanzhong, located at the middle of a straight line linking the two nipples. The lower Dantian is at the acupoint Qihai, which is 5cm below the navel or at the point 4.3cm below the navel. When diabetic patients do Qigong exercise, they should usually make the mind concentrate on the point 4.3cm below the navel.

Mechanism of Qigong Therapy

As an important constituent of TCM, Qigong is based on the

theories of TCM.

1. Qigong can reinforce the primordial Qi and strengthen the body resistance against diseases

The implications of Qi in TCM is very extensive. To put it briefly, Qi refers to both material and functional factors. It is the material foundation for all life activities as well as the functional manifestation of the physiological activities of the viscera. For example, the air breathed and the essence of food are the fine materials needed to nourish the whole body while the primordial Qi, chest Qi, nutrative Qi, defensive Qi and Qi of the five solid organs (the heart, liver, spleen, lung and kidney) and the six hollow organs (the gall bladder, stomach, small intestine, large intestine, urinary bladder and three Jiao), are the functional manifestations of the human body.

Qi is subdivided into the inherited and acquired. The primordial Qi belongs to the former while the chest Qi, the food essence, the nutrative Qi, defensive Qi and the visceral Qi belong to the latter. The primordial Qi, also known as genuine Qi, is inherited and stored in the gate of life. The primordial Qi acts as the motivating force to start a life process. The chest Qi, a combination of air in nature and essence gained from the digestion of food by the spleen and stomach, plays the role of stimulating the heart to pump blood and the lung to distribute nutrients. The nutrative Qi is derived from the essence of food. It circulates in the blood vessels to nourish the whole body and is involved in hemogenesis. The defensive Qi comes from Kidney Yang and is distributed all over the body surface to keep the Yang inside the body on one hand and defend the body against exopathogens on the other hand. Endowed with congenital Qi and dependent on the food essence, the Qi of the internal organs brings the functions of every organ into play. It is not difficult to see that every kind of Qi in the body has its own particular function and the primordial Qi plays a key role. It is regarded as the root of life. A man's health condition is decided by its prosperity and decline. When the primordial Qi is abundant, all the acquired Qi can be supported by it and thus there is good coordination among the viscera and a man remains physically and mentally healthy. On the contrary, if the primordial Qi is congenitally deficient or hurt by postnatal factors, all the acquired Qi would fail to be supported by it to become weak. As a result, the body is liable to various diseases.

In a sense, Qigong is a method for strengthening the body resistance and eliminating pathogenic factors to prevent diseases and preserve health. This, to some extent, is achieved by strengthening and nourishing primordial Qi through Qigong practice. "On How to Keep Innate Vitality Qi", a chapter in *Plain Questions* points out: "If you remain nonchalant to fame and gain, the genuine Qi will be with you; if you keep the spirit inside, how can diseases come about?" This is a brilliant exposition to and summerization of Qigong's mechanism in reinforcing and nourishing primordial Qi. In TCM, the essence of life, vital energy and mental faculties are considered the internal factors, which are the generalization of body functions. Qigong is a life-preserving method by which a practitioner trains himself through a combination of dynamic exercise of muscles, bones and skin in the exterior, and static exercise of essence of life, vital energy and mental faculties in the interior. The so-called "essence of life" consists of two parts: the congenital kidney essence and acquired food essence. Before the birth of a human being, it is endowed with the essence of its parents which develops into its body. After birth, the inborn essence of life is stored in the kidney to form the material basis of life. However, inborn essence of life depends on the nourishment by the acquired essence of food. Then the inborn essence and acquired essence are distributed all over the body by the heart, lung and spleen to enable the human body to carry out such physiological activities as growth and reproduction. Qigong produces a remarkable influence and effect on the essence of life. As long as a practitioner conducts Qigong practice in a proper way and with perseverance, Qigong can reinforce and replenish both the congenital and acquired essence of life. For instance, in case of the disturbance of digestive function, through the Qigong method of coordination between the heart and kidney, Kidney Yang can be consolidated and stored, Spleen Yang can be reinforced to function well and the Stomach Yin is nourished by the Kidney Yang. Thus the stomach can function well to make the food move along and the spleen can transform and transport nutrients properly. As a result, the blood vessles are filled with essence of food. This is good evidence of Qigong's effect on the essence of food. Qigong can also enrich the inborn congenital essence of life, which is stored in the kidney. The Qigong method of mind concentration on Dantian and the gate of life is just a way to enrich the kidney with the essence of life. The inborn essence of life has to be nourished by the acquired essence; through Qigong training and character molding of few desires, the acquired essence will become abundant and well stored, which will nourish the inborn congenital essence of life in the kidney to make it more consolidated. The consolidation of inborn essence of life will, in turn, lead to abundance of primordial Qi. This is an inevitable outcome of "training the essence of life to make it transform into Qi". It is evident that the effects of Qigong to increase essence of life and consolidate the kidney is the mechanism of Qigong to reinforce and nourish primordial Qi. In turn, the abundance of primordial Qi will motivate the internal organs to carry out normal and efficient physiological activities, which are also of great significance in the maintenance of health and defence against diseases.

2. The ability of Qigong in regulating Yin and Yang.

In TCM, maintenance of the normal vital activities of the human body is thought of as the result of the relative balance between Yin and Yang. "Grand Discussion on the Concept of Yin and Yang", a chapter of *Plain Questions*, says: "An excess of Yin leads to disorder of Yang and vice versa. An excess of Yang brings about heat syndromes and excess of Yin, cold syndromes." It is stated here that the imbalance between Yin and Yang means diseases. "On Adaptation of the Human Body to Natural Environment", a chapter in *The Yellow Emperor's Internal Classic*, says: "When dissociation of Yin and Yang occurs, the vital essence ceases to exist." It is pointed out in these statements that when an excess or a deficiency of either Yin or Yang reaches a certain limit, the relative equilibrium and unity relationship of Yin and Yang will be broken. Worse still, dissociation of Yin and Yang will occur, which will lead to near death state due to exhaustion of the essence of life. This is a form of transformation from the generation of disease to death. The form of transformation from a disease to recovery is also in conformity with the laws of balance between Yin and Yang. This is just what is referred to in the saying that "Yin and Yang in equilibrium bring about the recovery of a sound mind." During Qigong practice, when one concentrates to keep the spirit inside the body, Yang will not leak out, the spirit will not wander out, and the mind and spirit are kept inside to coordinate well with the kidney. This is the right way to consolidate Yang and replenish essence of life. During Qigong practice, concentrating on Dantian or the gate of life means the heart-fire goes down to the kidney. Thus the Kidney Yang can be warmed and Kidney Yin tonified. The method of concentrating the mind on Dantian is, therefore, in conformity with the principle of "consolidating Yang and replenishing the essence of life". When the kidney essence is abundant, the Kidney Yang will be plentiful enough to go up to the heart and nourish the Heart Yin. When the Heart Yin is nourished, the Heart Yin and Kidney Yin will be able to check the Heart Yang and keep the heart-fire from hyperactivity and running out. Thus the Heart Yang will go down to join the kidney even more easily. In this way not only the Yin is reinforced and the kidney essence protected, but through the replenishment of the Kidney Yang, both the Heart Yang and Kidney Yang are strengthened physiologically, which goes on to warm the Kidney Yin. When the Kidney Yin is not cold, the transformation of Qi from the kidney essence will be kept continuous. The coordination between the heart and kidney is very helpful in curing diseases and health conservation. The kidney contains two substances—kidney essence and Kidney Qi. The former is of the Yin nature, so it is also called primordial Yin or genuine Yin. The latter is of the Yang nature and is also known as primordial Yang or genuine Yang. Kidney essence nourishes all organs of the body while the Kidney Qi warms them and helps them to perform physiological activities. Heart and kidney stand for Yin and Yang. The coordination between the heart and the kidney is a brief generalization of the balance between Yin and Yang. The effect of Qigong on balancing Yin and Yang is achieved by coordination between the heart and kidney. Bringing about the balance between Yin and Yang is the theoretical basis of Qigong in curing diseases and conserving health.

Modern experimental research and clinical observations have also proved that a regulatory action of Qigong on the equilibrium between Yin and Yang exists widely. It is believed in TCM that the configuration and essence may transform into functions, which is a normal physiological phenomena showing that Yang originates from Yin. However, hyperfunction of the body may lead to consumption of the configuration and vitality. When one becomes tranquilized in Qigong practice, the excitability of sympathetic nerves is attenuated, body metabolism is lowered, hyperaction is corrected and hyperfunctioning is regulated. These are the concrete manifestations that Qigong can check Yang and reinforce Yin. Furthermore, it has been observed that in those who are classified as suffering from a deficiency of Kidney Yang according to the theory of kidney deficiency, after Qigong practice, the four cold limbs feel warm, the ketosteroid in urine restore to a normal level, the content of adenosine triphosphate, and cyclic adenosine monophosphate in plasma are increased, and the phagocytic power of white blood cells is strengthened. All these demonstrate Qigong's effect of reinforcing Yang. In short, the action of Qigong in regulating the dynamic equilibrium of Yin and Yang is achieved by "checking the hyperactive and reinforcing the hypoactive", and this action is shown on different levels. This is another aspect of Qigong's mechanism in treating diseases and preserving health.

3. The effects of Qigong in removing stagnation and obstruction in channels and collaterals and harmonizing Qi and blood

Channels and collaterals are chiefly connected with the transportation of Qi and blood, nourishment of the whole body, connection of the viscera with one another, and transformation of pathogenic factors, and are helpful in the diagnosis of diseases, message transmission, etc. They are of some guiding significance in physiology, pathology and treatment. When the channels and collaterals maintain normal physiological structures and functions, Qi and blood circulate smoothly in them, the solid and hollow viscera are in good condition, body and limbs are strong and vigorous. When there are pathological changes in structures and functions, the channels are often obstructed marked by Qi stagnancy and blood stasis, disharmony between the viscera, exhaustion of the nutrative Qi, weakness of the defensive Qi, and pains in the limbs. It is obvious that the channel and collateral system has much influence on the health of the body. One of Qigong's effects in curing diseases and conserving health is achieved by "removing the stagnation and obstruction in the channel and collateral system and harmonizing Qi and blood". Clinically, it has been observed that in patients with obstruction in the channels and collaterals and disharmony between Qi and blood, the determination values of channels and collaterals on the two sides of their body are not equal or differ very much, but after Qigong practice, they tend to be equal or the difference lessens considerably. The determination of Qi and blood demonstrated that those who are suffering from deficiency of Qi and blood can make themselves strong through Qigong exercises. The phenomena that channels and collaterals can conduct senses and Qi circulates in the Ren and Du Channels and other collaterals have also been observed during Qigong practice. These are all manifestations of Qigong's action in clearing stagnation and obstruction in channels and collaterals. In addition, a well-trained Qigong practitioner is able to "concentrate on a part of the body with Qi arriving at the same part simultaneously". According to the theory that "Qi is the commander of blood and when Qi is in smooth circulation, blood will also circulate well". In the part of the body or an internal organ where Qi goes, circulation of Qi and blood there is bound to increase. This is how Qigong can remove obstruction from the channel and collateral system and harmonize the Qi and blood to prevent and treat diseases.

4. Qigong cures and prevents diseases from the point of view of wholism

The concept of wholism is the guiding ideology of TCM theories. None of the basic TCM theories such as Yin-Yang theory, viscera theory, channel and collateral theory, Ying and Wei theory, embody this conception. The traditional theory and practice requirements of Qigong also reflect the conception of wholism that man corresponds to the universe. People who are good at preserving health also pay great attention to the regularity of daily life. Holding that the regularity of daily life should be adjusted in view of the changes of the seasons. "In the spring months", as they advocated, "one should go to bed early and get up early to have a good walk in the courtyard. In the summer months, one should also go to bed early at night and get up early and should not dislike sunlight. In the autumn months, one is to go to bed early and get up as early as chickens. In the winter months, one is to go to bed early at night but should not get up until the sun rises. They also advocate that spring and summer are the time for replenishing Yang while autumn and winter are the time for strengthening Yin." Health preservation through Qigong exercises is such a comprehensive regimen that not only attention should be paid to the training of an individual's internal factors but emphasis should also be laid on a comprehensive adjustment in "mind cultivation, changes with the seasons, regular daily life, and refraining from over-exertion". The mechanism of Qigong in the prevention and treatment of diseases is realized by maintaining and improving the equilibrium state of "correspondence between man and universe".

To sum up, the mechanism of Qigong in the treatment of diabetes consists of nothing more than these aspects. It is believed in

TCM that the pathogenesis of diabetes has the following features: ① The cause of the disease is deficiency of Yin and the manifestation is dryness-heat. The viscera affected are mainly the lung, stomach and kidney with kidney being the key organ involved. However, although pathological changes may be seen mainly in one of the three organs, they interact with each other in most cases. For instance, if the lung is in trouble due to dryness and deficiency of the Lung Yin, the lung fails to spread out body fluid. As a result, the stomach will fail to be nourished, and the kidney will lose the source of fluid nourishment. On the other hand, the hyperactivity of heat in the stomach would dry the lung fluid and consume the Kidney Yang. When the Kidney Yin is deficient, hyperactivity of fire will develop and flare up to hurt the lung and stomach. As a total result, dryness in the lung, heat in the stomach and kidney deficiency may exist concurrently. ② When these pathological changes develop further, they will lead to the impairment of Qi and Yin and deficiency of both Yin and Yang. It is from the conception of wholism or organic conception of human body that Qigong is employed in the treatment of diabetes because Qigong can reinforce the primordial Qi, bring Yin and Yang to balance, remove stagnation and obstruction in the channels and collaterals and harmonize Qi and blood to remove dryness and heat, increase body fluid and cure the disease by removing its causes. In addition, according to modern medical research on Qigong's physiological effect, Qigong exerts remarkable regulatory effects on the nervous, respiratory, digestive, circulatory and endocrine systems. The research on the endocrine system, in particular, shows that Qigong exercises can considerably augment the 17-ketosteroid. The mechanism is probably related to Qigong's regulatory effect on the hypothalamus-pituitary-adrenal reaction system. Besides, it has been observed that the content of cortical hormone in plasma varies notably before and after Qigong exercise. When a diabetic patient becomes tranquilized during Qigong practice, the vagus nerve is excited to stimulate the secretion of more insulin which will speed up the synthesis of hepatic glycogen and decrease the decomposition of hepatic glycogen to bring down the concentration of blood sugar. All these have provided a reliable scientific basis for the treatment of diabetes with Qigong.

Present Situation and Advances of Qigong Therapy in the Treatment of Diabetes

In order to make further study of the therapeutic effects of Qigong on diabetes, some medical research institutes have made clinical observations in recent years. It has been proved that Qigong therapy does have good therapeutic effects on diabetes.

Li Caiyan and others of Beidaihe Qigong Convalescent Home in Hebei Province treated 20 diabetic patients with a comprehensive therapy that the patients take Inner-nourishing Qigong as the main treatment along with some proper physical exercises such as shadow boxing and walking. A course of treatment lasts one month. One of the 20 patients received 4 courses of treatment, 1 received 3 courses, 12 received 2 courses, 3 received 1.5 courses, and 3 took only 1 course. The results were as follows: The treatment was very effective in 2 cases, accounting for 10%; 17 patients showed improvement, accounting for 85%; and 1 patient did not respond to the treatment, accounting for 5%. The total effectiveness rate was 95%. Shen Jizhou, Shi Binghe and so on of the No. 106 Hospital and No. 88 Hospital of the Chinese People's Liberation Army cooperated in determining the changes in blood lipid levels, blood sugar values, plasma insulin content, insulin release index and C-peptide of 20 diabetics before and after they practiced Crane Flying Qigong. The result of their observation showed that Qigong has a definite hypoglycemic effect. The blood sugar values on an empty stomach and half an hour after glucose intake dropped significantly. The average blood sugar values of the 20 cases before conducting Qigong practices were 10.93mmol/L(196.8mg%) on an empty stomach and 16.95mmol/L

(305.1mg%) after sugar intake. After Qigong exercises, they were 6.89mmol/L (124.0mg%) and 13.33mmol/L (239.9mg%) respectively. The determination results also demonstrated that Qigong has a blood-lipid lowering effect. Its cholesterol lowering effect is much stronger than its triglyceride lowering effect. The blood-lipid lowering effect and blood sugar lowering effect showed no difference. This indicates that Qigong has a reliable effect in lowering blood sugar. It was also observed in experiments that in 18 diabetic patients with decreased or roughly normal insulin release, their insulin release index of per oral glucose tolerance test on an empty stomach and 2 hours after glucose intake rose notably after being given Qigong treatment. All these results indicate that Qigong exercise have some effect in promoting the target cells' utilization of glucose. The physiology department of Chongqing Medical College made observations on the changes in blood sugar values of 5 hypertensive patients before and after they did Relaxation and Tranquilization Qigong. The average blood sugar value before Qigong practice was 7.24mmol/L (130.4mg%) and after practice, 5.41mmol/L (97.38mg%), the difference between the two values being 1.84mmol/L (33.03mg%) and the sugar-lowering rate being 25.24%. Geng Si of the No. 2 Construction Company of Taiyuan City in Shanxi Province reported that 3 diabetic patients practiced Yinshizi Quiet Sitting Qingong under his personal guidance. Significant effect was achieved in all of them. The blood sugar value before Qigong practice in one of them was 12.11mmol/L (218mg%) with glucose in the urine being positive (++++). After three months' practice of Qigong, his blood sugar concentration reduced to 6.39mmol/L (115mg%) with no glucose found in his urine. The patient was brought under clinical control. The Affiliated Hospital to Shanghai Medical University reported laboratory results of blood sugar determiation in 36 diabetic patients before and after one session of Qigong practice. In 29 out of 30 determinations, the blood sugar level decreased by varying degrees. The blood sugar level of 16 cases decreased from 12.32mmol/L (221.7mg%) before Qigong practice to 8.95mmol/L (161mg%) after practice. Of the 36 patients, those who persisted in Qigong practice, lowered their blood sugar levels in varying degrees after Qigong practice. They felt that symptoms such as thirst and asthenia improved greatly. The Shanghai Hypertension Research Institute treated 16 cases of hypertension associated with diabetes with Qigong therapy on the basis of diet control and relatively constant administration of hypoglycemic agents. The results showed that there was notable improvement in clinical symptoms, and blood sugar levels decreased from 9.51 ± 0.87mmol/L (171.25 ± 15.66mg%) before Qigong treatment to 8.39 ± 0.38mmol/L (151 ± 14.91mg%) after treatment. This revealed a significant difference ($p < 0.01$). Before Qigong treatment, the results on urosaccharometry were: 8 cases (+++ to ++++); 7 cases (+ to ++) and 1 case (+). After treatment, the results on urosaccharometry changed to: 4 cases (+ to ++); 8 cases (+) and 8 cases (−). The above evidences show that Qigong therapy does have a good curative effect on diabetes.

Wang Xiufang and so on in Lanzhou Air Force Hospital of the Chinese People's Liberation Army made initial research into Qigong's influence on the insulin levels in pilots. The subjects for this study were 12 randomly choosen male pilots aging 21-40, who practiced Dongyi Qigong conscientiously under the guidance of trainers both in the morning and evening. Before Qigong practice, determination of insulin levels was made and it was made again three months later. The insulin levels in these pilots decreased remarkably and the P value of the comparasion of the results was between 0.005-0.01, which is of great significance. The result shows that Qigong exercises can bring changes to the activities of the human autonomic nervous system and reduce the secretion of insulin. This is beneficial to the decomposition of glycogen and fat and increase of the contents of blood sugar and fatty acids.

It can be seen from the above mentioned research that Qigong does have a two-way regulatory effect on insulin, blood sugar, etc. Blood sugar can be lowered after Qigong practice. However, it is still unknown through what way Qigong takes effect in the treatment of diabetes. Future study should be focussed on the factors which influence glycometabolism to further reveal the mechanism of Qigong in the treatment of diabetes, and to find out the best Qigong practicing method so that Qigong can play a better role in clinical work.

Contents and Methods of Qigong Therapy in the Treatment of Diabetes

The history of treating diabetes with Qigong can be traced back to more than 1 000 years ago. In *General Treatise on the Causes and Symptoms of Diseases* compiled by Chao Yuanfang, a famous physician in the Sui Dynasty, treating diabetes with Qigong method special for diabetes was described. In recent years, Qigong therapy for diabetes has been popularized and employed gradually. Satisfactory therapeutic effects have been achieved. Now we recommend the following Qigong exercises which have proved effective in practice.

1. Inner-nourishing Qigong

(1) Posture: Usually latericumbent lying, supine lying or plain sitting posture is adopted.

(2) Respiration:

① The first respiration method: Close the mouth naturally and breathe through the nose. First inspire and lead the inhaled air down to the lower abdomen consciously. Do not exhale the air immediately after inhalation but hold the breath. After a pause, breathe out the air slowly. The breathing can be illustrated as inhaling—pausing—exhaling. Silent speaking of Chinese characters, phrases or simple sentences can be practiced at the same time as respiration. As a rule, silent speaking should begin from three-character phrases. Phrases or sentences of more words can be used step by step but usually no phrase of more than 9 Chinese characters should be used. The phrases or sentences chosen for this must denote relaxation, tranquilization, nice, healthy, etc., such as "*zi ji jing*" (Tranquilize myself), "*tong shen song jing*" (Relax the whole body and tranquilze the mind), "*zi ji jing zuo hao*" (Sit silent by myself), "*nei zang dong, da nao jing*" (Motivate the internal organs as if they were moving but tranquilize the mind), "*jian chi lian gong neng jian kang*" (Persistent Qigong practice is beneficial to health), etc. These silent speaking must be combined closely with the movement of the tongue. Take the silent speaking of "*zi ji jing*" for example. On inspiration, speak *zi* silently; during the pause of respiration speak *ji* and on expiration speak *jing*. Speak the rest following this as an example. The movement of the tongue refers to its up and down movements. On inhalation, the tongue rises up against the hard palate. During the pause it does not move and with expiration it lowers.

② The second respiration method: Breathe with the nose or both the nose and mouth. First inhale and then exhale slowly without any pause in between. The respiration pattern can be illustrated as inhalation—exhalation—pause. Silent speaking of words should also be done as in the above method. On inhalation, speak the first character, on exhalation, the second, and during the pause the third. The tongue should rise up against the hard palate on inhalation, lower on exhalation, and remain still during the pause. Repeat this cycle again and again.

③ Mind-concentration method: It is better to concentrate the mind on the lower Dantian. In Inner-nourishing Qigong, Dantian is said to be 5cm below the navel, at the acupoint Qihai. It was believed by the ancient Chinese people that the acupoint Qihai is the source where Qi is generated and a place where Qi is accumulated. However, the mind concentration here does not necessarily mean that it is on an accurate spot, but rather one should imagine Dantian as a round area on the surface of the lower abdomen with the acupoint Qihai as the center, or visualize it as a sphere-like body inside the lower abdomen. This Qigong exercise, rediscovered and sorted out by Liu Guizhen and so on, is suitable for all types of diabetics to practice. Generally, one should practice for

20 minutes both in the early morning and at night. Of course, the practice span can be lengthened according to one's own circumstances.

2. Six-character Qigong method

The six characters are selected in this Qigong practice because their pronunciations are identical with the nature of six solid and hollow viscera.

(1) Practice with the character *si*: Stand with the feet parallel, the knees slightly bent, the body tilting slightly forward, the abdominal muscles relaxed, the arms raised above the head, the palms obliquely upward on the forehead 1-2 fists apart. On inhalation, speak *xi* silently and on exhalation, speak *si* silently.

(2) Practice with the character *chui*: Stand with the feet parallel and apart as wide as the shoulders. Raise the arms up above the head from the sides of the body with the wrists crossed over the head. At the same time, inhale and speak *xi* silently. Then slowly bend the knees into a full squat. Lower the arms slowly from the front with the wrists crossed to hold the knees loosely with the elbows. At the same time, expire and speak *chui* silently.

(3) Practice with the character *xu*: Stand upright with the feet close together. Raise the arms from the sides of the body to a level position with the palms downward. Raise the heels with the big toes touching the ground forcefully. Open the eyes to gaze into the distance. The whole posture looks like a brave eagle soaring in the sky. On inhalation speak *xi* silently and speak *xu* on exhalation.

(4) Practice with the character *ke*: Stand with the feet parallel to each other and apart as wide as the shoulders. Raise the arms over the head from the sides of the body with the wrists crossed at the top. At the same time breathe in air and pronounce *xi* silently. Then bend the knees slightly and with the wrists still crossed, lower the arms to the lower abdomen from the front. Meanwhile relax the whole body, exhale and pronounce *ke* silently.

(5) Practice with the character *hu*: Stand with the feet parallel

to each other and apart as wide as the shoulders. Raise the arms above the head from the front with the palms against each other. Breathe in air and speak the word *xi* silently. Then twist the waist to the left and make the hands into fists. Rest the palmar side of the right fist gently on the acupoint Zhongwan and the palmar side of the left fist gently on the cartilage ribs of the left side. Meanwhile form the lips into an "O" shape, expire slowly and speak the word *hu*. Erect the body, raise the arms above the head from the sides with the palms against each other. At the same time inhale and speak *xi*. Twist the waist to the right, make the hands into fists, rest the palmar side of the left fist gently on the acupoint Zhongwan and that of the right fist on the right cartilage ribs. Meanwhile form the lips into an "O" shape, expire slowly and speak *hu* silently. Repeat the steps by turning the body to the left and right, 6 times each.

(6) Practice with the character *xi*: Take the supine lying position in which it is easier to perform abdominal breathing well to achieve the effect of regulating the three Jiao. Speak the word xi silently on inspiration. Expiration should be lengthened properly with the whole body relaxed and then speak the word *xi*.

The six-character Qigong method should be practiced 3 times a day, i.e. in the morning, at noon and at night, or practiced together with inner-nourishing Qigong. For patients with excessive internal heat, expiration should be longer than inspiration. Diabetes involving the upper Jiao is chiefly caused by deficiency of the lung, so it is advisable to do more practice with the character *si*; diabetes involving the middle Jiao is due to stomach troubles, so it is better to have more practice with the character *hu*; diabetes involving the lower Jiao is caused mainly by kidney disorders, so it is preferable to have more practice with the character *chui*. Qigong practice with the character *xu* benefits the liver, with the character *ke* benefits the heart, with *hu* strengthens the spleen, with *si* moistens the lung, with *chui* reinforces the kidney and with *xi* promotes the circulation of Qi in the three Jiao. On the basis of the above analysis, the Qigong practice with six characters should be performed under the guidance of a doctor with due attention to the excess or deficiency syndrome concerning the viscera, Qi, blood, Yin and Yang and according to the theory of five evolusive elements.

3. *Yinsizi* Quiet Sitting method

(1) Posture: Sit on a bed or a stool, take off the coat, and take single knee crossing posture, double knee crossing posture or free knee crossing posture. Overlap the hands with the palms upward and the right one on top. Rest them on the thighs and close to the lower abdomen. Sway the trunk to the left and right for 7-8 times and then sit with the body upright and with the nose in a vertical line with the navel. Open the mouth to let out the dirty air in the abdomen and then inhale fresh air slowly through the nose and mouth for 3-7 times. After that, close the eyes, keep the upper lip and teeth in touch with the lower, and the tongue up against the hard palate. After a long period of sitting, the body may tilt forward, backward or sideward. In that case, timely adjustment should be made. At the end of the quiet sitting, open the mouth to breathe out deeply for a dozen times so that the heat in the body can diffuse. Then gently shake the body, shoulders, neck and head in turn, and relax the feet and hands slowly. Rub the backs of the two thumbs together until there is a hot sensation and then rub the eyelids with them. Also close the eyes and rub the two sides of the nose with them. Rub the two palms until they are hot and massage the helixes with them. Finally, pat the head, chest, abdomen, back, arms, legs, feet and the soles with the palms before moving freely.

(2) Regulation of the respiration: Regulate the respiration to be very slow, gentle and even. Counting the numbers from 1-10 along with respiration may also be used again and again.

(3) Regulation of the mind: Try to attain mental concentration and eliminate distracting thoughts. When he tries to regulate his mind to concentrate, a beginner usually tends to remain absent-minded because he is either distracted by too many thoughts to concentrate or is so befuddled as to become sleepy. It is better for

him to forget about everything and concentrate only on the middle of the lower abdomen. In this way, he can be tranquilized gradually. Those who tend to be befuddled may try to pay attention to their nose tip to cheer up a little, or keep on counting numbers along with respiration to unify the mind and respiration. In this way both the absent-mindedness and the befuddleness can be avoided.

The best time for this Qigong exercise is *zi* time period (23 p.m.-1 a.m.) and *yin* time period (3-5 a.m.). It should be done in a clean room 3-4 times a day, 30-40 minutes a time. If one persists in this exercise, the stagnation and obstruction can be removed from all the channels and collaterals all over the body so that Qi and blood can circulate smoothly in the body, Yin and Yang can coordinate well, and a good therapeutic effect can be ensured in the treatment of diabetes. On average, a good result can be seen after one month's training and control of all symptoms can be attained after 3-4 months' practice. However, even after diabetes is brought under control, the patient should keep on the exercise for 20-30 minutes every day to make the effect permanent.

4. Special *Daoyin* Qigong for diabetes

(1) Preparatory exercise: Select a good place, such as woods in a park. Get up at half past six. Stand with the feet apart as wide as the shoulders and bend the knees slightly, not to exceed the tip of the toes. Draw in the chest, erect the back, relax the shoulders, droop the arms, erect the neck and head and place the soles firmly on the ground. Try to stop being restless and whimsical and get rid of all distracting thoughts to leave nothing in the mind. First practice stump-like standing and counter-abdominal respiration, leading the Qi by the mind down to Dantian first, next to the acupoint Changqiang, then into the Du Channel, up to the acupoint Baihui, into the Ren Channel, past the acupoint Queqiao to the acupoint Yongquan. Keep the Qi travelling round and round in this route and breathe 4 times a minute until a hot mass-like sensation generates in the lower abdomen (i.e. around Dantian), and then a hot sensation in the kidneys, back, testes,

the medial side of the thighs, the center of the soles and till all over the body. It takes about 20-25 minutes.

(2) Four-section stump-like standing Qigong for regulating the five solid viscera:

① Section 1: Coordination between the heart and kidney. Stand firmly like a stump. Lift up the arms and hands with the arms curving medially. Let the finger tips of the two hands come close to leave only a gap of less than 3.3cm in front of the lower Dantian so that the curved arms form a circle. Inhale in the process. Then move the arms apart outwardly with the palms facing laterally and exhale at the same time. When the hands are near the two acupoints Huantiao, turn the palms to face medially and rest them on the two Huantiao points. Repeat the movements 9 times.

② Section 2: Regulation of the liver and lung. Begin with stump-like standing. Lift up the arms and hands to the front as if holding something up and inhale at the same time. When the hands come to the acupoint Shanzhong, put the palms together as Buddhists do. Then while exhaling, slowly stretch the arms laterally and horizontally to the left and right with the fingers erected and palms facing sideward. Finally, while inhaling, return the arms to the original position like a wild goose setting on the ground. Repeat the movements 9 times. When the movements of Sections 1 and 2 are completed, stand still like a stump for 10-15 minutes.

③ Section 3: Strengthening the heart and spleen. Begin with stump-like standing. While inhaling, bend the waist leftward and backward, raise the right hand as if to prop up the heaven. Lift up the left foot to stand only on the right leg as a rooster often does. Then, while exhaling, draw with the right hand a circle from the top of the head to the left foot with the palm facing outward. Finally, return to the starting position along with inhalation. Now bend the waist rightward and backward, raise the left hand as if to prop up the heaven. Lift up the right foot to stand only on the left leg. Then the left hand draws a circle from the top of the head to the right foot with the palm facing outward along with proper breathing. Repeat the movements 9 times.

④ Section 4: Nourishing Yin and strengthening the kidney. Begin with stump-like standing. While inhaling lift up the hands from the lateral sides of the legs to the acupoint Shanzhong with the palms facing upward. Then while intorting the arms, flexing the wrists, turning the palms upward again, and exhaling, raise the arms high to form a circle. Then while inhaling and bending the back and waist, lower the hands and arms until the finger tips touch the ground. Finally, return to the starting position. Repeat these movements 9 times altogether. When the movements in sections 3 and 4 are completed, stand still like a stump for 10-15 minutes.

(3) Practice Taiji Quan (shadow boxing) two times.

(4) Shaking and swaying method: Begin with stump-like standing. Then step the left foot forward to shift the body weight on it. Raise the heels to stand on the tips of the feet, with the first two toes held to the ground firmly. Sway the arms to the left and inhale in the meantime. Then lower the heels and exhale in the meantime. Step the right foot forward. Raise the heels to stand on the tips of the feet. Raise the arms from the chest. Separate them to the left and right like a flying phoenix, and inhale through the nose in the meantime. Then flex the legs to squat with the hands resting on the knees while exhaling. Stand up and return to the original posture. Repeat the above actions for 9 times altogether.

(5) Perform shadow boxing with a sword two times and finally direct all the Qi to Dantian by the mind and end the whole set of exercise.

The special Daoyin Qigong for diabetes, develped through constant trials and errors in clinical practice, is an epitome of many schools of Qigong. If a diabetic patient adopts this Qigong series and perseveres in practicing it, notable effect can definitely be achieved. It takes about 40-50 minutes to complete the whole set consisting of the five kinds of exercises described above.

5. Genuine Qi circulating method

Step 1: As soon as the posture for Qigong practice is ready, narrow the field of vision, concentrate and pay attention to the nose tip for a short while. Then close the eyes to visualize the pit of the stomach. Listen to the sound of exhalation to keep it from becoming too coarse. While exhaling, concentrate on the pit of the stomach but let it be natural during inhalation. Repeat time and again as above and the genuine Qi will accumulate in the pit of the stomach. Keep on this exercise once in the morning, at noon and at night, doing it each time for 20 minutes.

Step 2: When the practitioner feels there is a hot sensation in the area of the pit of the stomach immediately he exhales after a period of training described in step 1, he should start practicing the skill of sending down Qi during exhalation to make Qi descend slowly and naturally to the lower abdomen—Dantian. Be sure not to be too eager for success, or there might be discomfort. It is required to practice three times a day, 20-30 minutes each time.

Step 3: When there is a hot sensation in Dantian through the training described in step 2, concentrate on Dantian and on the respiration. Three practice sessions should be conducted every day, 30-40 minutes each session.

Step 4: When the genuine Qi has accumulated at Dantian to a certain level to form a certain amount of energy, the Qi will ascend along the spinal column. Concentration should also go upward along with the ascending force without any distraction. If the Qi travels to a place and stops there, do not force it up because the speed of ascending of Qi depends upon the sufficient force in Dantian. Do not be too eager to make Qi go through "passes", but let it be natural instead. When the Qi goes up to the acupoint Yuzhen and cannot pass through it, just press the head top and it will pass through. At this stage, there should be more practice sessions a day, each to be prolonged to 50-60 minutes.

Step 5: In principle, it is still required to concentrate on the lower Dantian at this stage; however, if there is moving force in the top of the head, the concentration may be on the upper Dantian, which can be decided flexibly. It is required to have three training sessions every day, 60 minutes or more each time.

The five steps of this method are in a progressive order and the prior one forms the basis for the next. Therefore, in the practice of this method, on one hand, one should follow the natural development to carry out the training flexibly; on the other hand, he should be patient and persistent in the practice, but should not practice according to his own preference. Only when the practice is in proper order, proceeds step by step, and is done with persistence, can good clinical results be procured.

6. The Eight-section Callisthenics

Section 1: Propping up the heaven with the palms to regulate three Jiao.

Starting posture: Stand with the feet close together or parallel and apart as wide as the shoulders. Look straight ahead, raise the tip of the tongue against the hard palate, breathe through the nose, relax the joints all over the body, droop the arms naturally on the sides with the fingers stretching, keep the trunk naturally upright, let the toes touch the ground with force and lift up the center of the soles. Stand in this posture for a short while to concentrate.

Movements:

(1) Raise the arms slowly and obliquely from the left and right to the top of the head. Interlock the fingers of the hands. Turn the palms upward. Hold up the palms as if to prop up the heaven, and lift up the heels at the same time.

(2) Place the arms in the original position and lower the heels on the ground.

Repeat the above actions many times. Breathe in while lifting up the arms and breathe out while lowering them.

Section 2: Draw a bow as if to shoot a vulture.

Starting posture: Stand upright with the feet close together.

Movements:

(1) Take a side step to the left, flex the leg to assume a "horse-

riding" posture. Cross the forearms in front of the chest with the left arm on the inside and the right on the outside. Look at the left hand, which is then changed into a fist with the forefinger pointing up and the thumb stretching out to form a "V" shape. Then the left arm pushes to the left and stretches out straight. Move the head to the left while moving the left hand and look at the forefinger of the left hand. Meanwhile, clench the right hand into a fist which pulls horizontally to the right as if drawing a bow.

(2) Resume the original posture.

(3) Take a side step to the right, flex the legs to form a "horse-riding" posture. The other movements are the same as in (1) except that the left and right are reversed.

(4) Return to the upright standing posture.

Repeat the above actions many times. Inhale while stretching out the arms and drawing "bow", and exhale while resuming the original posture.

Section 3: Regulating the spleen and stomach by raising a single arm.

Starting posture: Stand upright with the feet close together or with the feet parallel and apart as wide as the shoulders and the arms drooped naturally.

Movements:

(1) Turn the right palm upward and raise it over the head. The fingers should be close together side by side with the tips pointing to the left. Meanwhile, turn the left palm to press downward with the fingers pointing to the front.

(2) Return to the original posture.

(3) All the movements are the same as in (1) except that the left and right are reversed.

(4) Return to the original posture.

Repeat many times. Inhale while raising the right palm and pressing down the left and exhale while returning to the original posture.

Section 4: Look around to treat five strains and seven impairments.

Starting posture: Stand upright with the palms pressing tight to the lateral sides of the thighs.

Movements:

(1) Turn the head slowly to the left to look back.
(2) Return to the original posture.
(3) Turn the head slowly to the right to look back.
(4) Return to the original posture.

Repeat many times. Inhale while looking back and exhale when returning to the original posture.

Section 5: Sway the head and buttocks to eliminate heart-fire.

Starting posture: Stand with the feet about three feet apart and flex the knees to assume the "horse-riding" posture. Rest the hands on the thighs with the part between the thumbs and forefinger facing the front.

Movements:

(1) Bend the head and the body deeply forward. Shake and sway them in an arch as much as possible in the left-front; meanwhile, sway the buttocks to the right. Stretch out the left leg and buttock properly to facilitate the swaying.
(2) Resuming the starting posture.
(3) The movements are the same as in (1) except that the left and the right are reversed.
(4) Return to the starting posture.

Repeat many times. Inhale while swaying and exhale while resuming the starting posture. The hands on the thighs may move with the swaying of the body.

Section 6: Pull the toes with the hands to reinforce the kidney and waist.

Starting posture: Stand upright with the feet close together.

Movements:

(1) Bend the body forward gradually with the knees straight and the arms drooped. Try to hold the toes with both hands (if impossible, just try to touch the ankles with the fingertips) and keep the head up a bit.

(2) Return to the starting posture.

(3) Place the hands on the back to hold against the back bone and gradually extend the body backward.

(4) Return to the original posture.

Repeat the movements many times and natural respiration is preferred during this section of the exercise.

Section 7: Clench fists and look with wide open eyes to build up strength and stamina.

Starting posture: Stand with legs apart and then flex the knees to form a "horse-riding" posture. Clench the hands into fists which are placed beside the waist with the palm side up.

Movements:

(1) Stretch the right fist slowly forward until the arm is straight with the palm side of the fist downward and look straight ahead with wide open eyes.

(2) Return to the original posture.

(3) Stretch the left fist forward in exactly the same way as described in (1).

(4) Resume the original posture.

Repeat many times. Exhale while stretching the fist and inhale while retrieving it.

Section 8: Rise and fall on tiptoes to dispel all diseases.

Starting posture: Stand upright with the palms pressing tight to the thighs.

Movements:

(1) Lift up both heels about 3.3-6.6cm above the ground and at the same time extend the head upward as if to prop up something with it.

(2) Lower the heels on the ground and return to the starting posture.

Repeat many times. Inhale while lifting up the heels and exhale while lowering them.

This set of callisthenics should be practiced 2-3 times a day. It is suitable for patients suffering from a deficiency of both Liver Yin and Kidney Yin, or a deficiency of both Qi and Yin.

7. Chao's Special Qigong Exercises for Diabetes

Step 1: Unbutton the clothes, loosen the belt, lie supine and keep the mind tranquilized. Then extend the waist to keep it in suspension with the back and sacral parts supporting the body. Place the hands naturally beside the body, drop the eyelids slightly, and raise the tongue against the hard palate. Take five deep, gentle, even and long breaths through the nose and bulge the lower abdomen with the rhythm of respiration.

Step 2: On the basis of the above posture, put the tongue tip in between the lips and teeth and move it from the upper jaw to the lower, from the left side to the right for 9 rounds, and then from the right to left for another 9 rounds. Then "gargle" 18 times with the saliva produced in the mouth during the tongue movement. Finally swallow the saliva slowly in several times and imagine being sending it to the lower Dantian. Thereafter, lie still for several minutes.

Step 3: Stand up and go out of the room. Walk slowly in a quiet place with fresh air and a lot of trees for 120-1 000 steps with a light heart.

This Qigong method is recorded in *General Treatise on the Etiology and Symptoms of Diseases* written by Chao Yuanfang. It is suitable for diabetics mainly involving the upper Jiao marked by thirst, polydipsia, difficulty in urinating, etc. The exercise should be done 2-3 times a day.

8. Teeth-knocking and saliva-gargling method

(1) Sitting still: Sit with erected back, neck and head, look straight ahead, draw in the chest, make fists by holding the thumb with other four fingers, place the fists on the thighs, raise the tip of the tongue to touch the hard palate loosely, droop the eyelids to visualize the viscera (i.e. to imagine as if one were seeing an internal organ), make inside listening, concentrate on the lower Dantian, relax completely and breathe naturally.

(2) Knocking teeth: When the practitioner is fully tranquilized and concentrating, he is to knock the upper and lower teeth with each other for 36 or 81 times at a slow and even rate.

(3) Tongue churning: Move the tongue against the upper and lower palates and the inner and outer sides of all teeth from the left to the right and then from right to the left for 9 or 18 times each. Do not swallow the saliva produced at this time.

(4) Saliva gargling: Close the mouth to blow out the cheeks and rinse the mouth for 9 or 18 times with the saliva produced during tongue churning.

(5) Swallow saliva: After gargling, swallow the saliva in three times, each time with some force. The swallowing often produces notable sounds. Then lead the saliva with mind down in the direction of the Ren Channel to the lower Dantian.

(6) Ending practice: Concentrate on Dantian for about 3-5 minutes. Then put the palms together and rub them until they are very warm. Rub the face with the warm hands, starting from the forehead, down to the sides of the nose and the lower jaw, and then up to the cheeks, the front of the ears and the temples, finally return to the forehead. Rub 9 times.

This Qigong method is able to strengthen Yin and replenish the essence to decrease the fire of deficiency type in the upper Jiao. *Essentials for Life Preservation* says: "One should often knock the teeth with the tip of the tongue to induce saliva because, when swallowed, it benefits the internal organs, beautifies skin, delays the aging process and prolongs life." The following can be found in *Talks on Medicine in Youyu's Study*: "In case one cannot go to sleep at night due to the flaring up of exuberant heartfire, he should bulge out his cheeks to produce a mouthful of saliva, and then swallow it in three times. Repeat the process several times and it will work because the reluxed saliva (a Qigong term for saliva produced during Qigong training) can check flaring fire." After bulging out the cheeks and gargling with saliva, the thirsty sensation in the mouth will die away immediately. This Qigong method is, therefore, a traditional health and life preserving method and a wonderful treatment for diabetes.

9. Other auxilliary treatments

(1) Yogism therapy: With regard to his or her own physical

condition, a patient may choose some yogism postures for exercise, such as supine lying, snake-shape lying, locust-shape lying, anteflexed latericumbent and semi-latericumbent lying, retroflexed latericumbent lying and supine lying with sprawling limbs, before or after Qigong pratice, or at some other time. If 3-4 kinds of them are choosen and practiced regularly, the symptoms are bound to be improved, the effect of Qigong training enhanced, and the diabetes brought under effective control.

(2) Patting the acupoints Shenshu and Mingmen: Stand relaxed and tranquilized, separate the two legs, bend down and make the hands into hollow fists to pat the areas of the acupoint Shenshu and Mingmen gently with even forces for 60-100 times. Then slowly stand upright and imagine that a moving Qi from the kidneys is circulating all through the body and all the sick and turbid Qi is emitted into the ground through acupoint Yongquan.

(3) Concentration of the mind on acupoint Yongquan: Constant concentration of the mind on the acupoint Yongquan will lead Qi downward. On inhalation, imagine as if the feet were inhaling. When standing or sitting, intentionally place the feet firmly on the ground; when lying, put the two soles together to rub each other frequently, or massage the acupoint Yongquan, Taixi, Kunlun and the toes with the hands.

Points for Attention in Qigong Therapy

1. To deepen the understanding of Qigong therapy

It is essential to have some basic knowledge about how to practice Qigong, to build up confidence in Qigong, to be determined to practice it and practice it with perseverance and concentration. After a proper Qigong method is chosen, keep practicing it regularly. Never play fast and loose or work by fits and starts.

2. Observe the principle of correspondence between man and the universe

(1) Choose a suitable environment for Qigong practice: The principle is to choose a place with fresh air and quietness and

peace. A place in the open country with flowers, plants and trees is most ideal. It is beneficial to health for a diabetic to practice Qigong near cypress or Chinese parasol trees but not near a dead or dying peach tree, tombs, and a place without fresh air. Do not practice Qigong under burning sun, in cold or strong wind, or when it is raining heavily, or when there is thunder and lightning.

(2) It is better to practice Qigong in the two-hour time periods of *zi* (11 p.m.-1 a.m.), *wu* (11 a.m.-1 p.m.), *mao* (5-7 a.m.) and *you* (5-7 p.m.) or in the six Yin time periods of *wu* (11 a.m.-1 p.m.) *wei* (1-3 p.m.), *xu* (3-5 p.m.), *you* (5-7 p.m.), *shu* (7-9 p.m.) and *hai* (9-11 p.m.) to nourish Yin and eliminate dryness.

(3) The direction of Qigong practice: In general, the practitioner should face the west, south, east or face the sun during the day and the moon at night. The direction may be chosen according to individual conditions. For example, choose the north to nourish the kidney.

3. The selection of Qigong method

Qigong practice should follow the principle of concurrence of training and nourishing, or integration of dynamic Qigong with static Qigong. Do not lay particular stress on either training or nourishing. Since there are differences in individual constitutions, disease conditions and types of disease among the diabetic patients, an individual patient should practice Qigong according to his or her actual condition under the guidance of his doctor. Of all the Qigong methods introduced in the previous section, Inner-nourishing method and *Yinshizi* Quiet Sitting method belong to static Qigong, by which one can nourish the primordial Qi and regulate the balance between Yin and Yang systemically. The patient should also select suitable exercises from the six-character Qigong to treat the three types of diabetes which involves the upper, middle or lower Jiao discriminatingly according to the five-evolusive-element theory and under the guidance of a doctor. Of the dynamic Qigong methods, the patient should mainly practice

Eight-section Callithenics selectively to regulate the corresponding internal organ, normalize the flow of Qi in the whole body, remove obstruction in the channels and collaterals and harmonize the Qi and blood. Also, all diabetics should practice teeth-knocking and saliva-gargling methods. If practiced regularly, they are able to nourish Yin, replenish life essence, and eliminate fire of deficiency type to produce good therapeutic effects on diabetes.

4. Practice of Qigong should be integrated with self-cultivation through meditation

Sun Simiao of the Tang Dynasty said in his *Prescriptions Worth a Thousand Gold*: "The principle of nourishing one's nature is not to walk too long, stand too long, sit too long, lie too long, listen too long and watch too long." He also wrote: "Those who are good at preserving their health usually try to have fewer thoughts, fewer concerns, fewer desires, fewer cares, fewer words, fewer laughters, fewer worries, fewer joys, fewer excitements, fewer rages, fewer likes and fewer bad deeds. These twelve 'fewer's' add up to a total foundation for self-cultivation." Diabetics should try to avoid the interference by strong emotions, and always keep an optimistic mind. Do not practice Qigong when one's mood is disturbed, such as overjoy, rage, or great sorrow, or when one is excessively hungry, overeaten or overtired.

5. Points for attention before and after a Qigong practice session

(1) Go to the toilet to relieve oneself. Unbutton clothes and loosen the belt. Wear a pair of flat-heel shoes. It is better to have a loose suit made specially for Qigong practice because overtightness of clothes may possibly hinder the normal flow of Qi.

(2) Twenty minutes before a Qigong practice session, the practitioner should stop vigorous physical and mental activities, such as running, jumping, boxing, chess, and playing cards, so that during Qigong training, the muscles all over the body are relaxed and the mind is set at rest. This is helpful for regulating respiration, becoming tranquilized and achieving mind concentra-

tion on Dantian.

(3) It is required to start and end Qigong training steadily. At the stage of ending a practice session, the practitioner must especially first practice concentrating on Dantian quietly for a while to conduct Qi to Dantian. Never end the practice hastily or stop abruptly to engage in something else.

6. The three "regulation's" must be fulfilled during Qigong practice

(1) Relaxation of the whole body must be achieved during regulation of postures. During a practice in standing posture especially the practitioner must loosen the clothes and belt, erect the head as if it were holding something on it, relax the shoulders, droop the arms, draw in the chest, erect the back, relax the waist and abdomen, draw in the hip, relax the knees, press the toes tightly on the ground, droop the eyelids to visulize the viscera, close the mouth and raise the tongue against the palate. It is especially important to raise the front part of the tongue against the hard palate, for only in this way can the Qi in the Ren and Du Channels be interchangeable.

(2) Before practicing Qigong, it is better to open the mouth and blow out air, imagining that the turbid air is flowing out of the body with the blowing. Then close the mouth and inhale fresh air three times. After that let the respiration be normal and regulate the respiration method gradually with the mind. The respiration must be in good coordination with the actions in the Qigong method so as to benefit the functional activities of Qi. The ultimate requirement for respiration exercise is to achieve a deep, long, even, and gentle mode of respiration. This can be achieved only through much respiration training but should not be sought after sedulously. To lengthen and force the respiration purposely should be avoided.

(3) The exercise of mind concentration must be coordinated with the exercise of respiration and posture. During Qigong practice, mind concentration should cooperate with the rising, lowering, opening, closing of postures. To exercise the mind concen-

tration, one should first of all have "faith" in the value of Qigong exercise. No matter what method of mind concentration one is practicing, it will lead to success through constant exercise. However, the practitioner should not be overeager for quick results. He should refrain from joy or anger, worry or panic when pictures emerge in the mind. Neither should he talk about them. He should adroitly conduct the exercise according to circumstances rather than pursue certain pictures in his mind sedulously.

(4) During the practice of Qigong, especially when the practitioner has become tranquilized, loud noises and shouts from people in the vicinity, or piercing and tremendous sound should be avoided because these abrupt provocations may frighten him to render him so nervous and scared that he could not but suspend the Qigong practice for a few days or even over ten days, and in a severe case the functional activities of Qi in the practitioner may be reversed or upset giving rise to Qigong-related problems. Therefore, when the practitioner reaches tranquilization and is subjected to drastic external provocations during Qigong practice, it is imperative for him to try his best to be in possession of himself. Should there be any trouble in the course of Qigong training, the practitioner should consult his doctor for help.

7. Qigong practice should be combined with dietary management

The daily diet should be a low-sugar diet consisting mainly of wheaten food. The patient should also have sufficient fresh vegetables, which can help ease the hungry sensation. Sugar-rich foods should be kept out of the diet to prevent the rise of blood sugar and aggravation of his condition.

Generally, after 7-30 days of Qigong training, therapeutic effects can be noticed, and after 3 months of Qigong training, remarkable effects will be produced. Usually a course of treatment with Qigong training lasts 3 months. At the initial stage of the course, drug therapy should be maintained. The dosage should be cut off gradually and finally stopped under the doctor's supervision and with the achievement of Qigong training. In addition, diabetic patients should also take part in some recreational and physical activities but overexhaustion should be avoided. They should not seek after the result of Qigong training seduously but should take Qigong training in an orderly way and advance step by step. Weak patients should prolong the practice session little by little rather than keep on a long session in spite of difficulty lest they should get more harm than good.

Acupuncture and Moxibustion Treatment for Diabetes

A Brief Account About Acupuncture and Moxibustion in the Treatment of Diabetes

The classic medical literature on the treatment of diabetes with acupuncture and moxibustion by all generations of medical scientists is still used to guide clinical treatment and scientific research.

The history of treating diabetes with acupuncture and moxibustion is very long. The following is recorded in *On Channels Written on Silk* unearthed in the Mawangdui No. 3 Han Tomb in Changsha of Hunan Province: "… for polyuria, polydipsia, … apply moxibustion to the Jueyin Channel." The work was proved by textual research to have been written earlier than *The Yellow Emperor's Internal Classic*. In "Collected Biographies of Bian Que and Cang Gong" in *Records of the Historian*, there are such medical case records of how Bian Que treated diabetes due to lung trouble: "It is diabetes due to lung disorder…. Apply moxibustion to foot Shaoyang Channel of the patient as well as the Shaoyin Channel…, and then give him Pinellia Pill to take." Bian Que advocated to treat the disease with both medicine and acupuncture. Huangfu Mi of the West Jin Dynasty wrote in his work *A-B Classic of Acupuncture and Moxibustion*: "For diabetes marked by fever, yellow complexion and eye, puncture acupoint Yishe; marked by polydipsia, puncture Chengjiang; marked by frequent eructation, aphasia due to Qi obstruction in the throat, cyanosis in the hands and feet, yellow urine, constipation, sore throat, spitting blood, hot sensation in the mouth, and saliva thick as glue, puncture Taixi. For diabetes due to deficiency of Yin Qi and heat in the Middle Jiao marked by polyrexia, hot sensation in the abdomen, irritability and ravings, puncture Sanli." This selection of different acupoints for different types of diabetes laid a foundation for the later generations of physicians to treat diabetes on the basis of differentiation of symptoms and signs to classify it into different types. In *Prescriptions Worth a Thousand Gold* and *A supplement to Essential Prescriptions Worth a Thousand Gold* written by Sun Simiao of the Tang Dynasty, there are many more detailed descriptions about the treatment of diabetes with acupuncture and moxibustion and combination of drug therapy and acupuncture treatment. For example, in Vol. 2 of *Prescriptions Worth a Thousand Gold*, this is written: "For diabetes marked by polyuria, it is effective to apply moxibustion to the small fingers of both hands and feet and the cervical vertebrae, then apply moxibustion to Jiejian in the middle of the backbone and two points of Yaomu. Also apply moxibustion to the spot 4cm below the acupoint Pishu on the back, two Shenshu acupoints and one Guanyuan point." *The Medical Secrets of an Official* written by Wang Tao of the Tang Dynasty also recorded the acupoints of moxibustion for treating diabetes. *The Illustrated Manual of Acupoints of Bronze Figure* compiled by Wang Weiyi of the Song Dynasty recorded many acupoints for treating diabetes. Included in *Experience on Acupuncture and Moxibustion Therapy* compile by Wang Zhizhong of the Song Dynasty was a special volume devoted to the treatment of diabetes with acupuncture and moxibustion. *The Understanding of Bian Que's Medical Experience* written by Dou Cai pays a great deal of attention to treatment of diseases with moxibustion, laying special emphasis on the significant effect of warming and tonifying primordial Yang in the treatment of diseases. There is a case record of diabetes in the book, which reads: "Diabetes was cured after 300 moxa-cones of moxibustion was applied to both Guanyuan and Qihai in association with administration of *Sishen Dan* (Pill from Four Marvellous Drugs) for 60 days." It can be seen from this that moxibustion along with medicine can ensure a better therapeutic effect. In *Great Compendium of Acupuncture and Moxibustion* by Yang Jizhou of the Ming Dynasty, many acupoints for treating diabetes and prescriptions of acupuncture treatment in verse were collected. In A *collection of Gems in Acupuncture and Moxibustion* compiled by Gao Wu, *A Great Collection of Acupuncture and Moxibustion* by Xu Feng, and *Illustrated Supplementary to Classified Canon* by Zhang Jiebin of the same dynasty, records of treating diabetes with acupuncture and moxibustion can be found. In the Qing Dynasty, *The Agglomeration of Acupuncture and Moxibustion* by Liao Runhong, *The Source of Acupuncture and Moxibustion* by Li Xuechuan and "Personal Insight of Acupuncture and Moxibustion", a chapter in A *Gold Mirror of Medicine* by Wu Qian, all recorded many acupoints and acupuncture prescriptions for diabetes. Although TCM and acupuncture and moxibustion made very slow progress in the period of Republic of China (1911‐1949), some scholars who devoted themselves to acupuncture and moxibustion continued to treat and prevent diseases with them for the working people. Mr. Cheng Dan-an (1931) from Wuxi of Jiangsu Province is the representative figure of them. In his *Revised and Enlarged Chinese Acupuncture and Moxibustion Therapy*, he recorded the treatment of three types of diabetes with acupuncture and moxibustion and emphasized that good therapeutic results could be obtained by integrating acupuncture with medicaments.

In the recent half century, rapid development can be seen in the undertaking of acupuncture and moxibustion and clinical and scientific research work in treating diabetes with acupuncture and moxibustion. There have been frequent reports on preventing and treating diabetes with acupuncture and moxibustion in monographs and treatises by medical scientists in the field. The representative works are *A Concise Edition of Science of Acupuncture and Moxibustion* compiled by the Research Institute of Acupuncture and Moxibustion under the TCM Research Academy, and *Therapeutics Volume of Acupuncturology* compiled by Shanghai College of TCM, both of them boast of prescriptions and methods for treating diabetes involving the upper, middle and lower Jiao with acupuncture and moxibustion. In terms of methods of acupucture and moxibustion treatment, many new methods have been invented on the basis of inheriting and carrying on the traditional ones, such as acupoint injection technique, auriculoacupuncture, acupoint magnetotherapy, nerve trunk stimulation therapy, plum-blossom needle (pyonex) and integrated acupuncture and massage therapy. Now acupuncture and moxibustion therapy has become one of the effective non-pharmacotherapies in the treatment of diseases. It has been observed in the application of this therapy that it boasts the following advantages: reliable effects, very little side effects and simplicity and convenience of application. The therapy has, therefore, been very popular among the diabetic patients.

Mechanism of Acupuncture and Moxibustion in the treatment of Diabetes

In the long clinical practice, medical scientists of both ancient and modern times have made a lot of brilliant expositions and have found many scientific proofs for the effects and mechanism of acupuncture and moxibustion in the treatment of diabetes. Particularly in recent decades, many new points of view have been advanced through clinical treatment and research. They are very important in expounding the mechanism of acupuncture and moxibustion.

1. Traditional understanding of acupuncture and moxibustion in the treatment of diabetes

(1) The differentiation of three types of diabetes and regulation of the balance between Yin and Yang in the viscera: The exposi-

tion of the causes, symptoms and treatment of diabetes in *The Yellow Emperor's Internal Classic* laid the foundation for the diagnosis and treatment of three types of diabetes involving the upper, middle and lower Jiao based on the overall analysis and differentiation of symptoms and signs. The expositions have yielded great influence on the treatment of diabetes in later times and are still effectively guiding today's clinical work of acupuncture and moxibustion. In the treatment of diabetes involving the upper Jiao, stress is laid on clearing away dryness-heat in the lung and promoting production of body fluids to ease thirst, for which purpose the acupoints Dazhui, Feishu, Yuji, Hegu, Taiyuan, Jinjin and Yuye are frequently used with uniform reinforcing-reducing needling manipulation. Dazhui and Hegu are punctured to clear the dryness-heat; Yuji, the spring point of the Lung Channel, is punctured to clear lung-fire, Feishu and Taiyuan, to remove dryness by reinforcing the lung and promoting production of body fluid. Quick punture of Jinjin and Yuye can not only clear away heat but also send up body fluid. The acupuncture of all these points can eliminate pathogenic heat, promote the production of body fluid, and hence the symptoms and signs of diabetes will vanish automatically. As for the treatment of diabetes involving the middle Jiao, the principle is to clear away the fire in the stomach, replenish Yin and promote the production of body fluid. The following acupoints are commonly used: Pishu, Weishu, Zhongwan, Zusanli, Neiting, Quchi and Hegu. Uniform reinforcing-reducing technique should be adopted during the acupuncture of Pishu, Weishu and Zhongwan while reduction method should be used during the acupuncture of other points. Puncturing Pishu, Weishu and Zhongwan is to regulate the functions of the spleen and stomach, to remove intense heat from them and promote the production of body fluid. Since both the stomach and the large intestine belong to Yangming Channel, acupoints Zusanli, Neiting, Quchi and Hegu of the hand Yangming Channel and foot Yangming Channel are punctured to remove the dryness-heat in the stomach and intestines and thus to ameliorate the symptoms of diabetes involving the middle Jiao. The principle of treatment of diabetes involving the lower Jiao is nourishing Yin and strengthening the kidney. The acupoints often used are Shenshu, Ganshu, Guanyuan, Sanyinjiao, Taixi and Rangu, punctured with reinforcing method. The effects of acupuncture of these points are: puncturing Shenshu and Ganshu replenishes Kidney Yin, puncturing Guanyuan consolidates the kidney and thus rectifies the deficiency of the lower Jiao, puncturing Sanyinjiao regulates Qi of the liver, spleen and kidney, and puncturing Taixi and Rangu of the Kidney Channel reinforces Kidney Yin and removes fire of deficiency type. The above mentioned prescriptions are just examples for the treatment of the three different types of diabetes involving respectively the upper, middle and lower Jiao, and the acupoints in the prescriptins are not immutable. The doctor may make flexible selection according to his own point selection habit. However, the general aim of treatment is removing the pathogenic heat and nourishing the body fluid in the viscera to achieve the balance between Yin and Yang of the viscera.

(2) Regulating Yin and Yang to rectify imbalance and disorder: There are these statements in the chapter "On the Origin and End of Channels" in *Miraculous Pivot*: "What is most essential in applying acupuncture treatment is that the doctor must know the importance of regulating Yin and Yang. Only when Yin and Yang are harmonious can the vital essence and energy be abundant and the physical body and vital energy be well united to house the spirit properly." In the human body, the Yin and Yang are interdependent. Although the pathological basis of diabetes is deficiency of Yin, protracted diabetes is apt to consume Yang and lead to deficiency of both Yin and Yang, so in the acupuncture treatment of diabetes, reinforcement of both Yin and Yang is advisable. The points for this purpose include Pishu, Shenshu, Mingmen, Qihai, Guanyuan, Zusanli, Sanyinjiao, Taixi, etc., and reinforcing method is usually used. In addition, mild-warm moxibustion with moxa stick or cone may be applied. The aim of puncturing Shenshu, Mingmen, Guanyuan, Taixi and Qihai is to

nourish Kidney Yin and reinforce Kidney Yang. By puncturing Pishu, Zusanli and Sanyinjiao, the spleen and stomach can be reinforced so that they will help strengthen the kidney in turn. The joint effects of these points and the combined application of acupuncture with moxibustion enable Yang to generate profusely by virtue of the consolidated Yin and enable Yin to find inexhaustible sources because of the invigoration by Yang. In case of deficiency of both Yin and Yang, strict sterile measures must be taken during acupuncture treatment to prevent infection because such patients have very poor body resistance and are apt to be infected.

2. Modern research on the action and principles of acupuncture therapy in the treatment of diabetes

In the recent four decades, scholars in China and abroad, on the basis of the experience in acupuncture and moxibustion gained by their forerunners and with the aid of related modern theories, have made a vast number of observations and a great deal of research on animals and human bodies in the action and principles of acupuncture and moxibustion in treating diabetes. They have come to the following tentative conclusions:

(1) Acupuncture has a regulating action to normalize blood sugar level. It has been found in animal experiments that after the test of influence of acupuncture on insulin and adrenalin secretion in animals with high blood sugar level, the high blood sugar level drop rapidly. On the other hand, puncturing some acupoints of animals with low blood sugar level, the blood sugar level quickly rises to normal. There is good ground to infer that acupuncture has the action to regulate the level of blood sugar and improve the body's mechanism of regulating blood sugar. These actions of acupuncture are obtained partly through the vagus nerve, and partly by increasing the sensitivity of glucoreceptors in β-cells to glucose, or possibly at the same time increasing the reactivity of peripheral tissues to insulin.

(2) Acupuncture has the actions of regulating the functions of vegetative nerves, rectifying endocrine dysfunction and restoring

the normal functions of islets. It is believed by some people that the development of diabetes is closely related to the dysinsulinism caused by functional disturbance of vegetative nerves. If sympathetic hyperfunction is present, the glands controlled by the sympathetic nerves will secrete absolutely or relatively more hormones that can increase blood sugar to be antagonistic against insulin, resulting in increase of blood sugar. On the contrary, if hypovagotonia is present to lead to insufficiency of insulin secretion and high blood sugar content, the failure of islet functions will take place as a result. Nourishing Yin and removing pathogenic heat is the fundamental principle in the treatment of diabetes. It is thought by some doctors that nourishing Yin is to stimulate the vagus nerve while removing heat is to inhibit the sympathetic nerve. It was also reported that acupuncture with "setting the mountain on fire" needling method can raise the blood sugar level while with "penetrating-heaven coldness" needling can lower the blood sugar level. But acupuncture with uniform reinforcing-reducing needling has little influence on blood sugar. It is demonstrated from these that different needling methods produce different actions on the body, especially on the functions of vegetative nerves, which bears direct influence on the rise or drop of the blood sugar level.

(3) Acupuncture acts on the central nervous system to promote the secretion of insulin and thus to lower the blood sugar level, or sets up a new focus of excitation which occupies a rather large area in the central nervous system to regulate, through mutual induction, the brain's stimulation-inhibition relationship and thus to upset the stimulating action of the pathologic factors of the diabetic patient to lower his blood sugar level.

(4) Acupuncture produces not only an intra-pancreas action but also an extra-pancreas one. After acupuncture, the receptor number of the target tissues grows, insulin antagonism is improved and peripheral tissues are stimulated to utilize more glucose and bring down the blood sugar level. It was found that in the blood rheological observations that acupuncture can also promote depoly-

merization of blood cells and decrease the viscosity of blood to improve blood supply to tissues and blood vessels, and indirectly regulate the disturbance of glycometabolism and fat metabolism, which are not only beneficial to diabetes itself but are very significant for its cardiovascular complications. Besides, after acupuncture, there are changes in the level of enkephalin and endorphin—endogenous opium-like substances (OLS) in the body. These substances have good preventive and curative effects for the complications of diabetes.

(5) Acupuncture and moxibustion can decrease the content of T_3 and T_4 in the blood, which suggests that acupuncture and moxibustion can decrease the content of thyroid hormone in the blood to reduce the absorption of sugar in the intestines and decomposition of glycogen, and they are, therefore, beneficial to decreasing blood sugar.

(6) It has been proved in experiments that acupuncture and moxibustion can strengthen the functions of insulin in glycogen synthesis, zymolysis and utilization by tissues and thus lower the blood sugar level.

Present Situation of Research on Acupuncture and Moxibustion in the treatment of Diabetes

It has been proved in the clinical practice of previous generations of medical practitioners that acupuncture and moxibustion have reliable curative effects, are simple and convenient to practice and have very few side effects in the treatment of diabetes. In order to further probe into their mechanism in the treatment of diabetes, medical scientists in both China and abroad have in the recent four decades done a great deal in clinical observations and basic experimental research. In this field China has always been in the lead.

In the 50s, Chinese medical researchers found through electric needle acupuncture on rabbits with purposely induced high sugar tolerance curve that acupuncture has the action of regulating and normalizing the blood sugar level. It was found in further studies that acupuncture with electric needles on the acupoint Baihui of rabbits produces a hypoglycemic effect, but acupuncture on the channel acupoints or acupuncture with electric needles of animals such as dogs and rabbits with normal blood sugar produces little change in blood sugar. Puncturing Zusanli and Baihui or puncturing with electric needles the sciatic nerve in dogs and rabbits with artificial hypoglycemia induced by injection of insulin caused a rise of blood sugar level in most cases. These experiments suggest that acupuncture and moxibustion or electric acupuncture have a two-way regulatory action on blood sugar and this action is related to the original blood sugar level. Acupuncture works to produce the mentioned effect not only through the vagus nerve but possibly by increasing the sensitivity of glucoreceptors of β-cells to glucose or at the same time increasing the reactivity of peripheral tissues to insulin.

In the 60s, Chinese researchers produced artificial diabetes model by injecting tetraoxypyrimidine (alloxan) into white rats and observed the morphological changes in the treatment of diabetes with acupuncture. After injection of tetraoxypyrimidine, acupoints Ganshu, Pishu, Shenshu, etc., were acupunctured. The result showed that the urine sugar content increased remarkably in the control group while only very little and transient sugar in urine was found in the group receiving acupuncture. When the rats were killed a week later, it was found that the hepatic glycogen in the control group decreased remarkably, and there was small focal necrosis in the liver, shrinkage of islets and notable necrosis of β-cells. However, the hepatic and pancreatic tissues of the group receiving acupuncture had hardly any difference from those in the ordinary animals. The study provided the histomorphological basis for the treatment of diabetes with acupuncture. The observations are 20 years earlier than the structures observed in the same way under electronic microscope reported by Watarin and so on of Japan at the 7th International Acupuncture and Moxibustion Conference in 1983. In the 24 cases of diabetes treated with acupuncture and moxibustion by Shanghai College of TCM, the treatment achieved notable effects in 50% of cases, 37.5% of the cases had some improvement, while in only 12.5% of patients, the treatment showed no effect. The blood and urine sugar content before and after treatment was also compared under the condition of free diet. In 21 cases, the sugar content was lowered, the lowest blood sugar level being 9.4mmol/L (170mg/dI). The diabetes research group in the internal medicine department of Beijing Xiehe Hospital gave 8 OPD diabetics plum-blossom needle treatment and chiropractic on the basis of comprehensive treatment. The result was desirable: not only the symptoms were relieved, but the mean blood sugar value dropped from 9.36mmol/L (168.5mg/dI) before treatment to 5.68mmol/L (102.3mg/dI) after treatment. What is more, during the follow-up stage, the patients' condition continued to improve and tended to be stable.

In the 80s, a group of 24 diabetics were admitted to a hospital for treatment and observation. The essential acupoints for the treatment were Pishu, Geshu and Zusanli while other acupoints were chosen on the basis of differentiation of syndromes and symptoms and according to the channel theory. For instance, in the case of excessive thirst and polydipsia, Feishu, Yishe and Chengjiang were also punctured; in the case of polyphagia, bulimia and constipation, add Weishu and Fenglong; in the case of polyuria, lumbago, tinnitus, vexation, tidal fever and night sweat, add Shenshu, Guanyuan and Fuliu; in the presence of listlessness, asthenia, disinclination to talk due to deficiency of Qi, diarrhea, fullness of head, and heaviness sensation in the limbs, also puncture Weishu, Sanyinjiao and Yinlingquan. Diet control was practiced along with acupuncture, and for a few cases with severe complications or those who were long-term dependent on oral hypoglycemic agents, the normal daily dosage was given as usual at the beginning, but as soon as acupuncture treatment began to take effects, the original dosage was reduced to half or abandoned completely. The result was broken down as follows: The treatment showed remarkable effect in 11 cases, accounting for 45.8%, good effect and improvement in 4 cases respectively, accounting for 33.4%, no effect in 5 cases, accounting for 20.83%. The total effective rate was 79.16%. In the 19 cases in which the treatment was effective, the mean value of blood sugar on an empty stomach before treatment was 17.15mmol/L ± 4.0 mmol/L (308.8 ± 72.1mg%), while the mean value after treatment was 8.93mmol/L ± 3.60mmol/L (160.8 ± 64.9mg%), the difference between the two amounting to as much as 8.22mmol/L (148mg%), which was very significant. Another 29 cases of non-insulin-dependent diabetes due to deficiency of both Qi and Yin were treated with acupuncture plus diet control. The acupoints used in the treatment were Hegu, Fuliu, Dazhui and Yuji with additional points of Zhongwan and Qihai for obvious asthenia. The needling manipulation stopped as soon as needling sensation was felt by the patients and the needles were retained for 20 minutes. The result of the treatment was analysed. In 11 cases there was remarkable effect, in 16 cases there was improvement and 2 cases did not respond to the treatment. After acupuncture treatment, 5 cases needed to continue the drug treatment but 24 cases stopped drug therapy. Thirst, bulimia, polyuria and asthenia were improved or disappeared. Fasting blood glucose concentration decreased significantly as compared with that before acupuncture treatment. The result exhibited notable difference according to statistical process ($P < 0.001$).

Shao Zhengyi and others of pharmacology department of Nantong Medical College reported the influence on the blood sugar produced by injecting zinc-containing insulin into the acupoint Neiguan of mice. In their observations, 60 mice which had not been fed for 24 hours were randomly divided into 4 groups: in one group insulin was injected into the acupoint Neiguan; in another group, insulin was injected intravenously; in the third group, zinc-containing insulin was injected into the acupoint Neiguan;

and in the last group, zinc-containing insulin was injected subcutaneously. Blood glucose value before insulin injection and 5 minutes after the injection in various ways was determined with a same method. The result revealed that the decreasing percentage of blood glucose 5 minutes after zinc-containing insulin injection into the acupoint Neiguan was distinctly greater than that of the other 3 groups ($P<0.01$ vs $P<0.05$). It was believed by the authors that the trace amount of insulin and zinc released from protamine zinc insulin (PZI) acting on an acupoint can produce remarkable hypoglycemic effect. There is the possibility that acupoint injection might replace subcutaneous injection of insulin or mixed preparation of common insulin and PZI, for PZI injection into acupoints has quick action or both quick and persistent action. Zhan Jianfei and so on of Jiangxi Province obtained the impression from their study in the treatment of diabetes with acupuncture and moxibustion that it is not by acting on only one single system that acupuncture cures diabetes. They thought that acupuncture not only has the function of regulating insulin at molecular level but also has the effect of regulating the central nervous system so that it can regain control over the area. Among these effects, the increased functions of target cell receptors of insulin (i.e. the combining power and affinity of receptors) after acupuncture may be one of the most important reasons. Wei Jia and so on of Jiangxi Province also discovered in their studies that non-insulin-dependent diabetics who still retain some function of endogenous insulin secretion respond well to acupuncture treatment but the insulin-dependent diabetics who lack this function respond poorly to the treatment. In the case of diabetic patients with hypersecretion of insulin, acupuncture can lower the insulin level and increase the insulin secretion index while in patients of hypoinsulinism, acupuncture can raise the insulin level and all specific values of insulin, denoting that acupuncture possesses a very powerful two-way regulatory effect also on diabetic patients who are not dependent on insulin. As an objective index for the evaluation of the therapeutic efficacy in the treatment of diabetes with acupuncture, insulin index is well worth recommendation. Generally, diet control cannot take the place of acupuncture treatment. All the acupoints to be used should be chosen in accordance with the channel theory and overall analysis of symptoms and signs, and with the aim of bringing balance between Yin and Yang in the viscera by regulating the deficiency of Yin or hyperactivity of Yang. It was also reported that on observations of blood rheological changes before and after acupuncture in 20 cases of diabetes, the blood viscosity and plasma viscosity of diabetics were found much greater than those of normal people, but after acupuncture, the blood viscosity was remarkably diluted. This suggests that the action of acupuncture on pathological changes of micrangia is not limited only to the biological changes of blood vessels, nerves and active substances, but also has a good efficacy in cell depolymerization and lowering blood viscosity. Zheng Huitian of Shanghai reported in 1983 that in the treatment of diabetic cystipathy with acupuncture, dynamic examination of the urine stream was used for observation, and intravesical pressure volume curve was found to have been restored to normal in most cases after acupuncture, which denotes that acupuncture is capable of making the detrusor urinae contract so that the intravesical pressure is increased and the bladder shrinks easily. With the uroflometry as the index, diabetic cystipathy was found to have made various degrees of improvement after acupuncture treatment.

In the recent ten years or so, many researchers in countries other than China have made extensive studies in the treatment of diabetes with acupuncture and moxibustion and have made some achievements which have attracted the attention of the world. Kioroshi Harumiyako and so on of Japan treated 54 cases of diabetes with acupuncture and moxibustion, with Zhongwan, Liangmen, left Guanmen, left Fuai, Ganshu, Pishu, left Sanjiaoshu and both left and right Zusanli as the main points. For patients on whose back scleroma could be felt, moxibustion on the scleroma was given for five moxa cones. For those with thirst, Quchi and

Lianquan points were also punctured. If there were lassitude manifestations, Shenshu and Dachangshu were also used. When retinopathy is also present, Taiyang and Fengchi were also used, and if cutaneous pruritus is present, Quchi, Fengchi and Zhubin were added. Fasting blood glucose concentration was used as the index of therapeutic efficacy: a decrease of 1.72mmol/L (31mg/dI) being considered remarkably effective and a decrease of 0.61-1.11mmol/L (11-20mg/dI) being considered effective. Altogether, 54 patients were treated, a remarkably effective result was achieved in 19 cases, an effective result in 7 cases, and 18 cases were kept on a stable condition. Hisazawa Munetsune and others of Japan probed into the relationship between the endocrine function of the pancreas and channels and acupoints by means of acupuncture and moxibustion. When they applied acupuncture and moxibustion on the 8 acupoints Zhongwan, Tianshu, Quchi, Taichong, Zusanli, Ganshu, Pishu and Diji, they found that the additional insulin secretion was remarkably increased in a diabetic individual. On this basis, they made further observation on the influence of a single acupoint acupuncture on insulin secretion, and found that acupuncturing Quchi or Diji with the needle retained for 30 minutes remarkably increased insulin secretion, but acupuncturing Zusanli did not bring much changes. In glucose tolerance test, it was found that the blood glucose level was lowered while insulin content in the blood rose notably. They believed that the influence of acupuncture and moxibustion on blood glucose may possibly be due to their stimulating action on the vago-insulin system. Romanian researcher Ionescu-Tirgoviste and so on discovered that acupuncturing the point Sanyinjiao in diabetics seemed to have produced a regulatory effect on insulin secretion of the pancreas which maintains normal physiological functions. Lin Zhongguo of Japan made observations of the influence of moxibustion on alloxan diabetes in rabbits. He divided rabbits weighing 1.8-2.2 kg into several groups of eight each. The first was the control group, injected only with tetraoxypyrimidine. The second group was given moxibustion on acupoint Pishu as well as alloxan injection. The third was given moxibustion on acupoint Weishu as well as alloxan injection. The fourth was given alloxan injection plus moxibustion on acupoint Zhongwan and the fifth was given alloxan injection plus moxibustion on acupoint Baihui. Monohydric tetraoxypyrimidine dissolved in normal saline was injected through auricular vein, 70mg/kg of body weight. Two hours after injection, moxibustion was applied, 5 moxa cones (as big as a pea) per acupoint, once a day for 7 consecutive days. Feeding was stopped 12 hours before blood collection and then blood glucose was assayed. The experiments showed that, compared with the control group, the blood glucose value in rabbits of group 2 (moxibustion on Pishu) and group 3 (moxibustion on Weishu) decreased ($P<0.05$), having statistical value. The blood glucose value in rabbits of group 4 (moxibustion on Zhongwan) decreased remarkably, ($P<0.01$), having significant statistical value. The blood sugar content in some rabbits of group 5 (moxibustion on Baihui) increased and others decreased, without statistical value. Lin came to the conclusion that it is a feasible method to treat diabetes with moxibustion. To sum up, acupuncture and moxibustion have notable effect in lowering blood glucose concentration in diabetics, and is a very ideal method for relieving their clinical symptoms.

Methods of Acupuncture and Moxibustion in the Treatment of Diabetes

1. Essentials of diagnostics

(1) The diagnosis of the disease can be tentatively made on the basis of such typical symptoms as polydipsia, polyphagia, polyuria and asthenia characterizing the disease plus the concomitant symptoms such as numbness of the limbs, weakness, menstrual disorder, constipation, itching of the skin and in the private parts.

(2) A detailed inquiry about the history of the illness should be made to collect such data as obesity, too much fat and sweet food, any mental factors and family hereditory history. Related labora-

tory tests should be ordered and a diagnosis can generally be established on the basis of clinical symptoms, positive result of urine sugar test, increased urine specification, and fasting blood glucose concentration exceeding 7.22mmol/L (130mg%).

(3) Attention should also be paid to the presence of any complication such as T.B., multiple sores or furuncles, hypertension, arteriosclerosis, cataract, peripheral neuritis, etc.

(4) Subdivide the disease into three types—diabetes involving the upper Jiao, involving the middle Jiao and involving the lower Jiao by distinguishing the principal from the secondary of the three "poly" symptoms. Diabetes involving the upper Jiao is characterized mainly by thirst and polydipsia, being ascribed to trouble in the Lung Channel. Diabetes involving the middle Jiao is marked chiefly by bulimia and polyphagia, being attributed to disorder in the Stomach Channel, while diabetes involving the lower Jiao is marked chiefly by polyuria, being attributed to the disturbance in the Kidney Channel.

2. Treatment

Medical scientists of the past generations have accumulated rich clinical experience in the treatment of the disease with acupuncture and moxibustion. Yang Jizhou of the Ming Dynasty, in particular, is still highly praised today by the medical world both in China and abroad because he, on the basis of summerizing the experience achieved before him, introduced the treatment of diabetes in which acupoints should be selected according to differentiation of three varied types of diabetes. In addition to his method, some modern clinicians have laid emphasis on the combination of choosing acupoints according to the type of diabetes with choosing points symptomatically.

In terms of therapeutic methods, in addition to the principal method of acupuncture, moxibustion, auricular needle therapy, hydro-acupuncture therapy, plum-blossom needle therapy, and comprehensive therapy by combining several methods have also been adopted. The combination of acupuncture and drug therapy may also be used, with the latter withdrawn gradually soon after therapeutic effects appear. Hereunder, however, our discussion will focus on the commonly used acupuncture therapy in which acupoints are chosen on the basis of differentiation of three types of diabetes. In clinical application of acupuncture, a doctor should determine if the disease is principally involving the upper Jiao, the middle Jiao or the lower Jiao, symptoms and signs are mainly due to heat in the lung, due to heat in the stomach or due to deficiency of the kidney, and on the basis of this analysis, contemplate whether the treatment should lay emphasis on moistening the lung, clearing away stomach heat or tonifying the kidney so that the choice of acupoints and needling manipulations can fit in well with a particular patient's case. As the disease is apt to develop complication of skin infections, special attention should be paid to skin disinfection during acupuncture treatment. Prior to inserting a needle, iodine tincture should be applied followed by rubbing with 75% alcohol solution to eliminate the iodine.

(1) Diagnosis and treatment based on overall analysis and differentiation of symptoms, signs, cause, nature and location of the disease.

① Diabetes involving the upper Jiao:

Chief symptoms and signs: Excessive thirst, polydipsia, dryness in the mouth, frequent urination with sweet urine, red margins and tip of the tongue with thin and yellowish fur, and full and rapid pulse.

Principle of treatment: Moistening the lung to clear away heat and dryness, and promoting the production of body fluid to relieve thirst.

Acupoints: Dazhui, Feishu, Yuji, Hegu, Taiyuan, Jinjin and Yuye.

Operation: The points prescribed above may be used alternately in two groups. Reducing manipulation is used on puncturing Dazhui, Yuji and Hegu while uniform reinforcing-reducing manipulation should be employed for Feishu, and Taiyuan. The needles should be retained for 20-30 minutes, to be manipulated every 5-10 minutes. Jinjin and Yuye should be punctured rapidly without retaining the needle.

Acupuncture the above points once a day or once every other day.

Effects of the prescription: Excessive thirst and polydipsia result from insufficiency of body fluid due to impairment of the lung by dryness-heat. Acupuncturing Dazhui and Hegu is to remove dryness-heat; acupuncturing Yuji, the spring point of the Lung Channel, is to eliminate the pathogenic fire in the lung; and by acupuncturing Feishu and Taiyuan, the lung is strengthened to produce more body fluid and remove dryness. The rapid puncture of Jinjin and Yuye, as the supplement to the above acupoints, can not only remove heat but also induce the body fluid to ascend. The combination of these points has the effects of removing pathogenic heat and promoting production of body fluid so that the excessive thirst diminishes automatically.

② Diabetes involving the middle Jiao:

Chief symptoms and signs: polyphagia, bulimia, gastric discomfort with acid regurgitation, dysphoria with smothery sensation, profuse sweat, emaciation, constipation, excessive urine which looks turbid and is sweetish, yellow and dry tongue fur, and slippery and rapid pulse.

Principle of treatment: Removing fire in the stomach and nourishing Yin to promote the production of body fluid.

Acupoints: Pishu, Weishu, Zhongwan, Zusanli, Neiting, Quchi and Hegu.

Operation: Uniform reinforcing-reducing method is used on acupoints Pishu, Weishu and Zhongwan while reduction needling for other points. The needles are retained for 30 minutes and the treatment is given once a day or every other day.

Effects of the prescription: The stomach is in charge of thorough decomposition of food. However, when there is excessive dryness heat there, food is too easy to be consumed in the stomach to result in frequent hungry sensation. Unfortunately, since the food is not actually utilized by the body, emaciation results. In the above prescription, Pishu, Weishu and Zhongwan are used to regulate the functions of the spleen and stomach, remove heat in the stomach and promote production of body fluid. Since both the stomach and large intestine belong to Yangming Channel and their Qi links up in the channel, therefore, in the prescription, Zusanli, Neiting, Quchi and Hegu of the hand and foot Yangming Channels are used to remove dryness-heat in the stomach and large intestine and relieve the symptoms of diabetes involving the middle Jiao.

③ Diabetes involving the lower Jiao:

Chief symptoms and signs: Polyuria with turbid creamy sweet urine, excessive thirst, polydipsia, lightheadedness, flushing in zygomatic regions, fidget due to deficiency, dreaminess, spermatorrhea, lassitude in the loin and legs, dry skin, skin itching all over the body, red tongue with little fur and thready and rapid pulse.

Principle of treatment: Nourishing Yin and tonifying the kidney.

Acupoints: Shenshu, Ganshu, Guanyuan, Sanyinjiao, Taixi and Rangu.

Operation: Acupuncture all the points with reinforcing method and with the needles retained for 20-30 minutes, once every other day.

Effects of the prescription: The kidney stores the essence of life. When the Kidney Yin is deficient and loses the power to reserve the essence of life, it fails to prevent it from flowing down. Also, because the liver and kidney have a common source, Ganshu and Shenshu are chosen to strengthen both the Liver Yin and Kidney Yin. Guanyuan is used to consolidate the kidney and correct the deficiency of lower Jiao. Puncturing Sanyinjiao can replenish Qi to the liver, spleen and kidney channels. Acupuncturing Taixi and Rangu of the Kidney Channel can nourish the Kidney Yin and send down fire of deficiency type. Puncturing all these points works to nourish the Kidney Yin and replenish kidney essence.

④ Diabetes due to deficiency of both Yin and Yang:

Chief symptoms and signs: polyuria with turbid creamy urine. In a severe case, the patient may discharge by urine every bit he drinks. Darkish complexion, haggardness, black and dry helixes, lassitude in the loin and legs, myasthenia and coldness of the limbs, impotence, whitish and dry tongue fur and deep thready weak pulse.

Principle of treatment: Tonifying both Yin and Yang.

Acupoints: Pishu, Shenshu, Mingmen, Qihai, Guanyuan, Zusanli and Sanyinjiao.

Operation: Acupuncture all of the above points with reinforcing needling plus mild-warm moxibustion with moxa stick or cone. The treatment is given every other day.

Effects of the prescription: In human body, the Yin and Yang are interdependent. Although deficiency of Yin forms the pathological basis of diabetes, the protracted diabetes is apt to consume Yang and a deficiency of both Yin and Yang develops in the end. The points Shenshu, Mingmen, Guanyuan and Qihai in the prescription are used to nourish the Kidney Yin and tonify Kidney Yang. Pishu, Zusanli and Sanyinjiao are chosen to strengthen the spleen and stomach, which will in turn reinforce the kidney. The combination of these points and the combined acupuncture and moxibustion treatment enable Yang to generate abundantly because Yin is consolidated and enable Yin to find inexhaustible sources because Yang is invigorated.

Complications and concomitant diseases are common in cases with a long course or without proper and timely treatment. Therefore, apart from the foregoing treatment, measures to deal with the concomitant diseases may also be taken. For instance, if palpitation develops, Neiguan, Shanzhong and Xinshu may be added to the prescription. For insomnia, Shenmen and Sanyinjiao may be used. When there is pain in the costal regions, and jaundice, acupoints Zhigou, Yanglingquan, Danshu, Riyue, Qimen and Ganshu may also be included. In case of stomachache, add Neiguan, Zhongwan and Zusanli. In case of constipation, also puncture Tianshu, Dachangshu, Zhigou and Zhaohai. If diarrhea is present, add Tianshu, Qihai, Pishu and Shangjuxu. In case of urodynia, frequent micturition and urgency of micturition, also select Pangguangshu, Zhongji, Yinlingquan, Xingjian and Taixi. If pruritus vulvae occurs, Qugu, Xialiao, Xuehai, Ligou, Zhongdu and Xingjian should also be incorporated. If blurred vision develops, add Zanzhu, Fengchi, Guangming and Taichong.

(2) Electric needle acupuncture:

Acupoints: Yishu (5cm lateral to the lower border of the spinous process of the 8th thoracic vertebra), Feishu, Pishu, Shenshu, Zusanli and Sanyinjiao.

Operation: Only 2-3 acupoints are chosen for treatment at a time. After the needles are inserted, needling sensation is felt by the patient and reinforcing-reducing manipulations are completed, the needles are connected to an electric acupuncture stimulator by wires. Dense wave electric current may be used for stimulation for 15 minutes, once every other day.

(3) Auriculoacupuncture:

Acupoints: Spots corresponding to the pancreas, the endocrine area, the lung, stomach, kidney, bladder, hunger point and thirst point.

Operation: Choose 3-4 points at a time for treatment. After routine disinfection, puncture with filiform needles to give moderate or mild stimulation and then the needles are retained for 20-30 minutes. The treatment is given once every other day. Buried needling in auricular points or auricular-seed-pressing therapy (A mung bean or seed of Vaccaria segetalis is taped tightly to a particular auricular acupoint and pressed once in a while to stimulate the point for therapeutic purpose) may be used, once every three to five days.

(4) Plum-blossom needle treatment:

Acupoints: Jiaji points of the 6th-12th thoracic vertebrae and of the 1st-5th lumbar vertebrae.

Operation: Puncture slightly or moderately with plum-blossom needles, 5-10 minutes in each treatment, once every other day, 10 times for a therapeutic course. The intensity of puncturing may be flexibly adjusted according to a patient's condition, age, health, etc.

(5) Acupoint-injection:

Acupoints: Feishu, Pishu, Weishu, Sanjiaoshu, Shenshu, Quchi, Zusanli and Sanyinjiao.

Drugs for injection: Injection prepared from Safflower (*Flos Carthami*), Chinese angelica (*Radix Angelicae Sinensis*) and Astragalus (*Radix Astragali seu Hedysari*), or normal saline or small doses of insulin.

Operation: Choose 2-4 points at a time and inject 0.5-2ml of drug solution into each point, once every other day. A course consists of 5 times of treatment.

3. Selection of acupuncture prescriptions by ancient and modern medical scientists

(1) Universal prescriptions for diabetes:

① For diabetes, puncture Wangu point. —From "Diabetes and Jaundice due to Overflow of Five Qi", Vol. 11 of *A-B Classic of Acupuncture and Moxibustion*

② For diabetes with a course of over 100 days, never give acupuncture and moxibustion treatment because they are likely to cause infection at the punctured point with constant discharge of exudate to result in abscess or furuncle which will lead to emaciation and death in the end. Care should also be taken to prevent any accidental wound. For diabetes at the initial stage, acupuncture and moxibustion treatment can be conducted according to the prescriptions. If moxibustion on the Yin-points has no effect, it is then advisable to apply moxibustion to Yang-points. —From "Diabetes", Vol. 3 of *Classic for Saving Lives with Acupuncture and Moxibustion*

③ For diabetes, puncture Shuigou, Chengjiang, Jinjin, Yuye, Quchi, Laogong, Taichong, Xingjian, Shangqiu, Rangu and Yinbai. If the diabetes is over 100 days, never treat it with moxibustion. —From "Nose and Mouth", a section in *Classic of Treatment with Miraculous Effects*

④ Diabetes and other diseases: The three types of diabetes

have different symptoms, i.e., involving the spleen, involving the middle Jiao, and involving the kidney. It is recorded in *Plain Questions*: "As the stomach is deficient, a *dou* (an old unit of dry measure for grain, equal to a little more than a peck or 1/4 of a bushel) of food for a meal cannot prevent the patient from being hungry; when the diabetes involves the kidney, even a hundred cups of drinks cannot stop the thirst and the sex life is not satisfactory. These are the so-called three types of diabetes. They are caused by dryness in the spleen. Puncture Renzhong, Gongsun (two points), Pishu (two points), Zhongwan, Zhaohai (two points), Zusanli (two points, to relieve increased appetite and excessive hunger), Taixi (two points, to improve unsatisfactory sex life) and Guanchong (two points).—From "Notes to the Eight Methods of Mr Dou Wenzhen", Vol. 4 of *Great Collection of Acupuncture and Moxibustion*

⑤ For diabetes, acupuncture Jinjin, Yuye and Chengjiang, and also puncture Houxue, Haiquan, Renzhong, Lianquan, Qihai and Shenshu. —From "General Principles of Treatment", Vol. 9 of *Great Collection of Acupuncture and Moxibustion*

⑥ For diabetes, acupuncture Shenshu and Xiaochangshu. — From "The Key Acupoints for Moxibustion to Treat Various Syndromes", Vol. 11 of *Illustrated Supplementary to Classified Canon*

⑦ For diabetes, acupuncture Chengjiang, Taixi, Zhizheng, Yangchi, Zhaohai, Shenshu, Xiaochangshu, and acupoint on the little finger or the small toes (i.e. the tip of the little finger and toe).—From Vol. 3 of *On Classic of Acupuncture and Moxibustion*

⑧ It is put forward in some books on acupuncture and moxibustion that diabetes can be treated by applying acupuncture and moxibustion to Shuigou, Chengjiang, Jinjin, Yuye, Quchi, Laogong, Taichong, Xingjian, Shangqiu, Rangu, Yinbai, etc.

⑨ For diabetes:
   Acupuncture and moxibustion are very helpful for diabetes,
   Listed below are the common acupoints:

Ganshu, Pishu, Mingmen, Zhongwan, Guanyuan Shenshu, Plus Sanyinjiao, Xinjian, Yongquan and Rangu.

For this disease, the acupuncture should be in moderate stimulation, and moxibustion should often be applied to Mingmen and Guanyuan. —From *Pithy Formulae for Treatment by Acupuncture and Moxibustion On Acupoints of the Fourteen Channles*

(2) Prescriptions for different symptoms and signs of diabetes:

① For diabetes marked by fever and yellow complexion and eyes, puncture Yishe; for diabetes marked by polydipsia, puncture Chengjiang; for diabetes characterized by aphonia due to obstruction of Qi in the throat, cyanosis in the hands and feet, yellow urine, sore throat, spitting blood, hot sensation in the mouth, and glue-like saliva, puncture Taixi. If it is marked by bulimia, polyphagia, fever in the abdomen, dysphoria and ravings, due to deficiency of Yin Qi and due to heat in the middle Jiao, Zusanli is indicated. For diabetes with jaundice marked by one foot feeling hot and the other feeling cold, protrusion of the tongue and dysphoria and feeling of distension and fullness, puncture Rangu. —From "Diabetes with Jaundice due to Overflow of Five Qi", Vol. 11 of *A-B Classic of Acupuncture and Moxibustion*

② For diabetes characterized by dry throat, apply moxibustion to the three Yishu points, 100 moxa cones each. The points are on the back, 3 *cun* lateral to the lower border of the spinous process of the 8th thoracic vertebra.

For diabetes associated with cough and dyspnea, apply moxibustion to Jueyin, for as many cones as the patient's age.

For diabetes marked by dry throat, apply moxibustion to Xiongtang for 50 cones and Taiyang Channel of the foot, also 50 cones.

For diabetes characterized by thirst and polydipsia, apply moxibustion to foot Jueyin Channel for 100 cones and Yangchi, 50 cones.

If it is marked by frequent micturition with scanty urine, inability to make sperm ejaculation, tell the patient to open his hands, put the palms together with the thumbs side by side and the thumb nails closely together. Apply moxibustion to the triangle of flesh formed at the joining border in between the root parts of the two thumb nails for three moxa cones. Apply moxibustion to the big toes in exactly the same way. The treatment is administered every 3 days. —From "Diabetes", Vol. 21 of *Prescriptions Worth a Thousand Gold for Emergency*

③ For diabetes: Shangqiu is the acupoint for treating diabetes involving middle Jiao marked by dysphoria; Yishe is the acupoint for treating diabetes marked by fever and sallow complexion; Chengjiang, Yishe, Guanchong and Rangu are used for treating diabetes with polydipsia; Yinbai for diabetes marked by polydipsia and excessive thirst; Laogong for diabetes with bitter mouth, thirst and anorexia; Quchi for diabetes with cold and fever; Xingjian and Taichong for diabetes with dry throat and excessive thirst; Yishe and Zhonglushu for diabetes due to kidney deficiency marked by difficulty in perspiration, inability of the back and waist to bend forward and backward, distension in the abdomen and pain in the costal regions; Duiduan for diabetes marked by yellow urine and dry tongue; Rangu for diabetes marked by protrusion of the tongue and dysphoria; Shuigou for diabetes marked by unlimited drinking and Yanggang for diabetes. —From "Diabetes", Vol. 3 of *Classic for Saving Lives with Acupuncture and Moxibustion*

④ For diabetes due to deficiency of the kidney, puncture Rangu, Shenshu, Yaoshu, Feishu and Zhonglushu. Pinch up the skin and muscle on either side of the spine, at the spot 3 *cun* lateral to the lower border of the spinous process of the 8th thoracic vertebra and apply moxibustion for three moxa cones. —From Vol. 2 of *The Agglomeration of Acupuncture and Moxibustion*

⑤ In recent years the acupuncture and moxibustion department of the Affiliated Hospital to Shandong College of TCM has conducted moxa stick suspension moxibustion to treat diabetes and has achieved remarkable effects. The points for moxibustion are: Weiguanxiashu (i. e. Yishu), Pishu, Zusanli plus accessory points in the proper channels chosen symptomatically. In case of polydipsia, excessive thirst and dry mouth, add Feishu, Yishe and Chengjiang; for polyphagia, bulimia and constipation, add Weishu and Fenglong; in case of polyuria, lumbago, tinnitus, vexation, tidal fever and night sweat, Feishu, Guanyuan and Fuliu are of choice; in case of listlessness, lassitude, diarrhea, fullness of head, heaviness and lassitude of the limbs and trunk, Weishu, Sanyinjiao and Yinlingquan are selected. Mild-warm moxibustion treatment should be employed in most cases and should go on until the skin around the acupoint reddens, but be sure that the moxa stick or cone is not too hot so as to prevent infection. Moxibustion is applied on each point for 10-15 minutes, once or twice a day, 12 times forming a therapeutic course. The department treated 34 cases altogether. Of all the patients, 14 cases showed remarkable effect, 10 of which were treated only with moxibustion. Good effects and improvement were achieved in 6 cases respectively, 3 cases of which were treated only with moxibustion and 3 cases were treated with combined therapy respectively. No effect was achieved at all in 8 cases.

⑥ The acupuncture and moxibustion department of the affiliated hospital to Shandong College of TCM also employed ginger-separated moxibustion, the moxa cone being 1.5cm in diameter, 2cm in height and 0.5g in weight. The ginger slice being 3-4mm thick and 2cm in diameter. The acupoints used were divided into 8 groups and moxibustion was applied to one of the 8 groups alternately. Group 1: Zusanli and Zhongwan; group 2: Mingmen, Shenshu and Pishu; group 3: Qihai and Guanmen; group 4: Jizhong and Shenshu; group 5: Huagai and Liangmen; group 6: Dazhui and Ganshu; group 7: Xingjian, Ahongji and Fuai; group 8: Feishu, Geshu and Shenshu. Moxibustion with 10-15 cones was applied to each point and it took about 150 minutes at each treatment. The treatment was given once every other day, 30 days constituting a therapeutic course.

Accessory points were also used symptomatically. For diabetes involving the upper Jiao, Jinjin, Yuye (both punctured),

Neiguan, Yuji and Shaofu were included; for diabetes involving the middle Jiao, Dadu and Pishu were added; for diabetes involving lower Jiao, Rangu and Yongquan were added. Throughout the moxibustion treatment, oral hypoglycemic agents were cancelled. Before treatment, the blood sugar was 8.33-13.8mmol/L (150 - 250mg%), with an average of 9.76mmol/L (175.6mg%). After the first course of treatment, the blood glucose level lowered in average by 2.05 ± 0.83mmol/L (36.9 ± 15.0mg%) ($P<0.05$). At the end of the second course, the blood glucose concentration lowered again by 0.44mmol/L (8mg%). After the two courses, if the blood glucose level of a patient was lowered by 0.83mmol/L (15mg%) or more, the treatment was regarded as effective, which was found in 8 cases. Another 3 cases showed no effect.

(3) Prescriptions for diabetes involving the upper Jiao:

① For diabetes marked by polydipsia, puncture acupoint Chengjiang. —From "Diabetes with Jaundice due to the Overflow of Five Qi", Vol. 11 of *A-B Classic of Acupuncture and Moxibustion*

② For a child suffering from polydipsia with sallow complexion, apply moxibustion of one cone as big as a wheat grain to the two Yanggang points, which are at the depression 3 *cun* lateral to the lower border of the spinous process of the 11th thoracic vertebra. —From Vol. 2 of *Yellow Emperor's Chart of Acupuncture and Moxibustion*

③ Once I received a patient who drank frequently but his thirst was not relieved. I told him that he was suffering from diabetes resulting from deficiency of Spleen Qi and Lung Qi rather than heat in the interior. He told me that he had taken six doses of drugs with cold property, and though his fever was relieved, he still felt thirst all the time, had the feeling of fullness in the chest and hypochondria, and dyspnea. I said to the man: "In your original syndrome, only the spleen and lung were injured. Now the drugs of cold property you've taken have hurt your primordial Qi as well, so the spleen and lung fail in their function of transportation, resulting in retention of water below the heart." I gave him moxibustion at once on acupoints Guanyuan and Qihai, 300 cones for each point. I also gave him *Sishen Wan* (Pill Of Four Miraculous Drugs) for oral administration. Sixty days later, normal production of body fluid was restored. Every medical book explains that the condition is due to intense heat in three Jiao and so drugs of cold property are recommended. As a matter of fact, such drugs will kill the patient sooner than swords. As a doctor, one must be cautious. —From *Bian Que's Medical Experience*

④ It is recommended in some medical book that diabetes involving the upper Jiao can be treated in the following way: Acupuncture Renzhong, inserting the needle 2 *fen* deep, retaining and twisting the needle for 1 minute. Puncture Chengjiang, inserting the needle 2 *fen* deep, retaining and twisting it for 2 minutes. Puncture Shenmen, inserting the needle 3 *fen* deep, retaining and twisting it for 2 minutes. Puncture Rangu, inserting the needle 3 *fen* deep, retaining and twisting it for 2 minutes. Puncture Neiguan, inserting the needle 3 *fen* deep, retaining and twisting it for 2 minutes. Puncture Sanyinjiao, inserting the needle 3-4 *fen* deep, retaining and twisting it for 2 minutes.

⑤ The main acupoints for diabetes involving the upper Jiao due to dryness-heat in the Lung Channel marked by polydipsia with normal urination: Feishu and Shenshu. Auxilliary points: Neiguan and Yuji. All the points should be punctured with reducing manipulation. —From *A Handy Book for Treatment of Common Diseases with Acupuncture and Moxibustion*

⑥ Diabetes involving the upper Jiao is characterized by hot feeling in the throat, excessive thirst and polydipsia. Principle of treatment: clearing away heat in the Lung Channel to normalize the production of fluid. Acupoints: Feishu, Yuji, Lianquan and Hegu. Effects of the points: Puncturing Feishu and Hegu with reducing manipulation can eliminate the heat in the upper Jiao to moisten the lung. Yuji is the spring point of the Lung Channel and puncturing it with reduction method can remove heat from the lung. Puncturing Lianquan can promote production of body fluid to arrest thirst. —From *A Concise Course of Acupuncturology*

⑦ Diabetes involving the upper Jiao is marked by red tongue with fissures, a sensation of being burnt by fire in the throat, excessive thirst and polydipsia day and night.

Treatment: Removing heat to nourish Yin and removing fire from the lung to replenish body fluid.

Prescription: Acupuncture Feishu, Shaoshang and Yuji with reducing manipulation; acupuncture Jinjin and Yuye to bleeding. Sanjiaoshu and Yangchi are supplemented with reducing needling.

Effects of the prescription: Puncturing Feishu and Yuji can eliminate fire from the upper Jiao; acupuncturing Shaoshang can purify Lung Qi and clear heat from all the viscera; puncturing Jinjin and Yuye to bleeding helps Qi and blood circulate smoothly so that the body fluid can be transported to the upper Jiao. Since diabetes is a condition which may involve the three Jiao, Sanjiaoshu and Yangchi are used to clear away the accumulated heat in the three Jiao. —From "Therapeutics" in *Acupuncturology*

⑧ In recent years, the acupuncture and moxibustion department of the Affiliated Hospital to Shandong College of TCM has combined acupuncture with medicaments in the treatment of diabetes. To treat diabetes involving the upper Jiao, their principle is to moisten the lung and clear away heat in the stomach. The points for the purpose were Shenshu, Fuliu and Neiting plus the modified prescription for diabetes.

(4) Diabetes involving the middle Jiao:

① Diabetes involving the middle Jiao: Secret prescription of moxibustion for diabetes. Modern medical men do not examine what are the causes of this disease and do not discern whether the disease is of an excess or deficiency nature before they prescribe tonics indiscriminatively for all patients, which only renders the disease incurable. What a pity! They hardly realize that diabetes is due to the accumulation of heat…. There is a marvellous moxibustion method for the disease. Tell the patient to erect both hands with the nails of the middle fingers cut off. Place a moxa cone of the size of a soybean on the tip of both fingers. Have two assistants light the cones simultaneously and blow them from time to time to keep the moxa cones burning bright. Also apply moxibustion to Taichong of the feet in the same way. The moxa cones are 5-6 *cun* high. Only when the four acupoints are burnt to form four small pits can the treatment be effective. Soon after treatment the patient will have appetite and the jaundice will disappear. Moxibustion should be applied to Baihui in much the same way to the fingers and toes. This method never fails. —From "On Dryness", Vol. 13 of *Supplements to Danxi's Experiential Therapy*

② For polyphagia and emaciation: Pishu and Weishu. —From the section "The Heart, Spleen and Stomach" in *Classic of Miraculous Effects*

For diabetes: Puncture acupoint Taixi. —From the section "Swelling Problems" in the same book

③ To treat diabetes involving the middle Jiao with acupuncture and moxibustion, it is important to regulate the stomach. It is recorded in medical classics that when the pathogenic factors are in the spleen and stomach, Yang Qi is in excess but Yin Qi is deficient, and therefore, there is heat in the middle Jiao to cause bulimia. In this case, apply moxibustion to acupoints Sanli. Medical classics also recorded that if the Qi in the foot-stomach Yangming Channel is hyperactive, the chest and abdomen feel hot, the stomach will become so hyperactive as to cause polyphagia and bulimia (hunger). The heat should be cleared and the hyperactivity should be rectified with reducing method. —From The "Miscellaneous Diseases", Vol. 5 of *Standards for Diagnosis and Treatment*

④ For diabetes involving the middle Jiao: Puncture Zhongwan, Sanjiaoshu, Weishu, Taiyuan and Lieque with reducing manipulation; if marked by polyphagia, emaciation, a mass beside the umbilicus, and abdominal pain, apply moxibustion to Pishu for from three to as many moxa cones as the patient's age. Also puncture Jiangmen, Qimen, Taibai and Zhongwan. —From *The Ag-*

glomeration of Acupuncture and Moxibustion

⑤ It is reported in medical literature that for diabetes involving the middle Jiao, acupuncture Zhongwan by inserting the needle 5 *fen* deep, retaining and twisting it for 2 minutes, Sanjiaoshu by inserting the needle 3 *fen* deep, retaining and twisting it for 2 minutes, Weishu by inserting the needle 3-4 *fen* deep, retaining and twisting the needle for 2 minutes, Taiyuan by inserting the needle 2-3 *fen* deep, retaining and twisting it for 2 minutes, and Lieque by inserting the needle 2 *fen* deep, retaining and twisting for 2 minutes.

⑥ Diabetes involving the middle Jiao: dryness-heat in the stomach marked by thirst, bulimia, emaciation, etc. Principal acupoints: Weishu and Zhongwan (acupuncture). Adjuvant points: Zhaohai and Neiting (acupuncture with reducing manipulation). —From a medical book

⑦ Diabetes involving the middle Jiao: polyphagia, bulimia, emaciation, spontaneous sweating and frequent micturition. Treatment: it is preferable to clear away heat in the stomach to regulate the middle Jiao. Acupoints: Quchi, Neiguan and Zusanli. The effects of the points: Acupuncture the three points with reducing needling can clear away heat in the stomach to regulate the middle Jiao.—From a medical book

⑧ Diabetes involving the middle Jiao: polyphagia, bulimia, emaciation, thirst, polydipsia, constipation and urine turbid as pigwash. The treatment principle is removing heat in the stomach to nourish the Spleen Yin. Prescription: Weishu, Zhongwan, Xiangu, Pishu and Shuidao supplemented by Sanjiaoshu and Yangchi. Puncture all these points with reduction manipulation. Effects of the prescription: Acupuncture Weishu, Zhongwan and Pishu with reduction method to clear away the fire in the spleen and stomach, Xiangu to eliminate the dryness-heat in the Yangming Channel, and Shuidao to eliminate both heat in Yangming Channel and the heat accumulated in three Jiao. The elimination of fire in the stomach will lead to spontaneous recovery of the Spleen Yin. The additional treatment on Sanjiaoshu and Yangchi can clear away the heat accumulated in three Jiao. —From a medical book.

⑨ The acupuncture and moxibustion department of the Affiliated Hospital to Shandong College of TCM treated diabetes involving the middle Jiao with a combined therapy of acupuncture and medicine to clear away heat in the stomach and nourish the kidney by puncturing Zhongwan, Neiting and Sanyinjiao and giving oral administration of *Shigao Zhimu Tang* (Decoction of Gypsum and Anemarrhena) with Coptis, Bamboo Shavings and dried Rehmannia.

⑩ The acupuncture and moxibustion department of the Affiliated Hospital to Shandong College of TCM has adopted ginger-separated moxibustion in recent years to treat diabetes and remarkable effects have been achieved. In the treatment of diabetes involving the middle Jiao, Pishu, Geshu and Zusanli have been picked as the essential points and adjuvant points are added on the basis of differentiation of symptoms and signs in different channels ···. For polyphagia, bulimia and constipation, Weishu and Fenglong are picked.

(5) Prescriptions for diabetes involving the lower Jiao:

① For diabetes marked by frequent micturition, give moxibustion on the tips of the small fingers of both hands and feet and the cervical vertebrae. Moxibustion should also be applied to one Jiejian point which is in the middle of the spine, and to two Yaomu points. Give moxibustion to a spot 4 *cun* below Pishu on the back. All these points should be given moxibustion for as many moxa cones as the patient's age. Apply moxibustion to two Shenshu points and Yaomu points, which are 3 *cun* below Shenshu and 1.5 *cun* lateral to the backbone on either side, Guanyuan and two other spots which are 2 *cun* apart from it on either side, and two Yinshi points, which are 3 *cun* below Futu on the edge of the knee. Or moxibustion may be given to the point Shenxi, which is described in *The Yellow Empewror's Internal Classic* as being 1 *cun* below Futu. The points Ququan, Yingu, Yinlingquan and Fuliu are very effective in checking polyuria without hurting Yang Qi. They are also believed to be good for enuresis. The points Taixi, Zhongfeng, Rangu, Taibai, Dadu, Fuyang, Xingjian, Dadun, Yinbai and Yongquan should be given moxibustion for 100 cones each. Altogether, 47 points on the back, abdomen and two feet should be treated, of which Shenshu, Yaomu, Guanyuan and Shuidao should be given 30 cones each for 5 days in succession, that is, 150 cones each point. Yongquan, 10 cones; Dadun, Yinbai and Xingjian, 3 cones each; and 7 cones for each of the rest. For every point a moxibustion treatment course consists of five days and the treatment should be stopped after three courses. If, after this treatment of the Yin points, the patient fails to recover, it is then advisable to shift the moxibustion treatment to the Yang points, which are on the surface of the feet, and also the points Feishu and Zhongfu, in the direction and order of the points in Channels. The number of cones are the same as for the Yin points.—From "Diabetes", Vol. 21 of *Prescriptions Worth a Thousand Gold for Emergency*

② Diabetes involving the lower Jiao: Acupuncture Rangu, inserting needle 3-4 *fen* deep, retaining and twisting it for 2 minutes; puncture Shenshu, inserting the needle 3 *fen* deep, retaining and twisting it for 2 minutes; puncture Yaoshu, inserting the needle 2 *fen* deep, retaining and twisting it for 2 minutes; puncture Feishu, inserting the needle 2-3 *fen* deep, retaining and twisting for 2 minutes; apply moxibustion to Zhonglushu with 3 cones.—From a medical book

③ Diabetes involving the lower Jiao: Due to deficiency and exhaustion of Kidney Yin marked by thirst, polyuria which is so severe that the patient discharges all that he drinks by urination, and emaciation. Essential acupoints: Xinshu, Shenshu, Guanyuan and Zhongji. Puncture all the points. Adjuvant points: Fuliu and Kunlun, acupuncture with reinforcing-reducing manipulation.—From a medical book

④ Diabetes involving the lower Jiao: marked by polyuria, sediment in urine, gradual development of darkish complexion, and turbid urine. It is not uncommon that the diabetes involves the three Jiao simultaneously. If such symptoms and signs as excessive thirst and polyuria are present, it is diabetes involving both the upper Jiao and lower Jiao. In case of polyphagia and polyuria, it is diabetes involving both the middle Jiao and lower Jiao, which often leads to emaciation, myasthenia of the limbs, itching of the skin and listlessness when it lingers for many days. If complicated by carbuncle on the back, the diasese is in a critical condition. The principle of treatment is tonifying the kidney and nourishing Yin. Acupoints: Shenshu, Fuliu, Taixi and Sanyinjiao. Effects: Acupuncture of Shenshu, Fuliu and Taixi with reinforcing method can tonify the kidney to correct the deficiency of Kidney Yin. Sanyinjiao is the point of intersection of the three foot Yin Channels and acupuncturing it with reinforcing method can nourish Yin. If two types of diabetes occur concurrently, proper points should be picked symptomatically. —From a medical book

⑤ Diabetes involving the lower Jiao: marked by inability to control urination, black and dry helixes, darkish complexion, creamy urine, dysphoria and polydipsia. The principle of treatment should be eliminating the fire in kidney and increasing kidney water. Prescription: Shenshu, Guanyuan and Shuiquan, all punctured with reinforcing manipulation; Rangu and Xingjian, both punctured with reducing manipulation, plus Sanjiaoshu and Yangchi, both punctured with reducing method. Effects of the prescription: Acupuncturing Shenshu, Guanyuan and Shuiquan with reinforcing manipulation can nourish the kidney to increase kidney water; Rangu is used to eliminate kidney-fire and Xingjian for eliminating liver-fire. Since diabetes is due to pathological changes in three Jiao, Sanjiaoshu and Yangchi are added to clear away the accumulated heat in three Jiao. —From a medical book

⑥ The acupuncture and moxibustion department of the Affiliated Hospital to Shandong College of TCM has combined acupuncture with medical management to treat diabetes involving the lower Jiao by nourishing Yin, tonifying the kidney and descending asthenic fire. The acupoints used are Guanyuan, Daimai and Rangu. The drug given is *Zhibai Dihuang Tang* (Decoction of Anemarrhena, Phellodendron and Rehmannia).

⑦ The acupuncture and moxibustion department of the Affiliated Hospital to Shandong College of TCM has introduced ginger-separated moxibustion to treat diabetes and has achieved wonderful effects. In the treatment of diabetes involving the lower Jiao, Pishu, Geshu and Zusanli are used as essential points supplemented by adjuvant points selected on the basis of differentiation of symptoms and signs and in accordance with the channels, e. g. for polyuria, lumbago, tinnitus, vexation, tidal fever and night sweating, Feishu, Guanyuan and Fuliu are also punctured.

4. Acupoints commonly used to treat complications of diabetes

For retinopathy, Taiyang, Fengchi, Tongziliao, Yanglao, Guangming and Taichong can be chosen.

For itching of the skin or vulvae, Quchi, Zhubin, Qugu, Diji and Sanyinjiao may be used.

For impotence and menstrual disorder, Guanyuan, Zhongji, Guilai, Ciliao, Sanyinjiao and Taixi are of choice.

For diabetic constipation, Tianshu, Qihai, Shangjuxu, Zhigou and Zhaohai can be selected.

For diabetic chronic diarrhea, Tianshu, Shangjuxu, Guanyuan and Sanyinjiao are of choice.

For diabetes with the complication of peripheral neuropathy, Quchi, Waiguan, Hegu, Baxie, Zusanli, Juegu, Sanyinjiao and Bafeng are of choice.

In case of diabetes associated with intracranial neuropathy, Dicang, Jiache, Yangbai, Xiaguan and Yifeng can be used to treat facial paralysis; Tinggong, Tinghui, Yifeng, Zhongzhu and Waiguan for acoustic neuropathy; Jingming, Zanzhu, Taiyang, Yuyao, Tongziliao and Hegu for oculomotor paralysis.

In case of early diabetic cystipathy, Qihai, Lieque, Zhaohai, Shuidao, Huiyang, Zhonglushu and Weiyang are of choice. Mingmen, Shenshu and Guanyuan can be given moxibustion, and Huiyang, Zhonglushu and Weiyang can be punctured.

Points of Attention In the Treatment of Diabetes with Acupuncture and Moxibustion

1. Have a good knowledge about the indications of acupuncture and moxibustion. The levis-moderate diabetes and type II diabetes (NIDDM Type), especially the obese type, respond well to acupuncture and moxibustion therapy while type I diabetes (IDDM Type), emaciated type and severe type of diabetes do not respond well to the therapy, for which reason, acupuncture and moxibustion therapy should not be used alone. Instead, it should be used cautiously or be avoided in the management of all kinds of acute or severe complications. It is forbidden in case of skin infection.

2. Most diabetics are constitutionally weak and insufficient in body resistance so that they are liable to infections, for which reason, prior to acupuncture and moxibustion treatment, strict disinfection of the area round the acupoint should be carried out and suspension moxibustion method is preferred so as to prevent any burnt to the skin which may cause infection.

3. If the patient has been treated with hypoglycemic agents or insulin injection before this therapy, the original dosage should be kept up at the beginning of acupuncture and moxibustion treatment. Only when the condition is improved can the dosage of medicine be cut off gradually or cancelled completely.

4. During acupuncture and moxibustion treatment, the diet should be controlled and dietotherapy should be integrated with this therapy. Physical exercises should be performed every day to build up the health, which can intensify the effects of this therapy and helps this therapy take quick effect.

Massotherapy In the Treatment of Diabetes

A Brief Account of Massotherapy

Massage is not only a very important component part of TCM, but also one of the important therapeutic methods of TCM. It is a therapy which needs no medicine but only the massagist's hands to apply treatment on the body surface according to different disease conditions and with different manipulations. It belongs to the category of external treatment. In history there have been many different terms referring to the therapy in Chinese, such as *anmo* (chirapsia), *anqiao*, *qiaomo*, *qiaoyin* and *anfu*. Massotherapy has been used to treat diseases for more than 2 000 years in China. According to *Descriptive Accounts of Books in Dynastic Histories* compiled in the Han Dynasty, the earliest monograph on massage was entitled *Ten Volumes on Massage by Yellow Emperor and Qi Bo*, which, to our great pity, was lost long ago. Fortunately, in the earliest medical classic extant in China, *The Yellow Emperor's Internal Classic*, there are already descriptions about massotherapy. For example, in the chapter "Qi, Blood, Configuration and Will" in *Plain Questions*, there is such description: "If a person is terrified times and again, obstruction in the channels and collaterals may develop to lead to numbness or apathy in the body and limbs, which can be cured with massage and wine preparations." Written in another chapter "On Different Prescriptions for One Kind of Disease" in *Plain Questions* are these statements: "The central areas are plain and damp. Therefore, they are suitable for all kinds of living things to live. However, the people living on them take many different things as food and do not exert much, so they often suffer from diseases marked by flaccidity with cold limbs, or fever and chills. These diseases should be treated with *daoyin* (a kind of Qigong) and *anqiao* (another ancient term for massage)." Here it is stated that diseases marked by flaccidity with cold limbs, fever and chills can be treated with massage.

The Spring and Autumn Period, Warring States Period, Qin Dynasty and Han Dynasty saw further development in massotherapy, which displayed a unique therapeutic effect. According to *Records of the Historian*, Bian Que, a most famous doctor of the Qin Dynasty, once treated the corpse-like syncope of the crown prince of Guo Kingdom and restored him to life, which became an interesting story on everybody's lips in the time. In the Sui Dynasty massage was used as a very popular therapy for diseases and was highly appreciated by the government circles as well as the medical circles. In the Office of Imperial Physicians of the Sui Dynasty, there was a special department of massage under the direction of two officials who were experts in massotherapy. In the Tang Dynasty, massage was more prevalent in the treatment of diseases. According to "Officials" in *The New Book About the Tang Dynasty*, "There was one official who was proficient in massage and four massagists who were commissioned as officials at or below the 9th grade in rank and were responsible for teaching the methods of *daoyin* (i. e. physical and breathing exercises) to treat diseases and set injuries and fractures." According to *Six Canons of the Tang Dynasty*, there were 56 people who were engaged in massage in the Office of the Imperial Physicians and fifteen of them were massage doctors. With the cultural exchanges between China and foreign countries during the most prosperous period in the Tang Dynasty, massotherapy was spread as one of the effective TCM therapeutic methods to Japan, Korea, France, etc.

In recent years, massotherapy has given better play to its unique effect in the treatment of diabetes. Massage can not only improve the symptoms of diabetes and lower the blood sugar level but also has good preventive and curative effects on the complications of diabetic microangiopathy and neuropathy. Moreover, Since massage does not have any side and toxic effects that frequently arise in pharmacotherapy in the treatment of diseases, does not need knives and needles, is simple and convenient to carry out, is safe and reliable with remarkable therapeutic effects, and can be used either for keeping physical fitness or treating diseases, it is very popular among the diabetics.

Mechanism of Massotherapy

It is believed in TCM that the viscera, channels and collaterals, Yin, Yang, Qi, blood and body fluids are the material basis of the vital activities of human body. The normal vital activites of the body are the results of the good coordination between viscera, channels and collaterals, Yin and Yang, Qi, blood and body fluids, among which the channels and collaterals play the most important role. They are bridges linking the internal and external activities of the viscera and are canals in which Qi, blood and body fluids circulate. When they are out of order, disharmony between different viscera and between Yin and Yang, and disturbance in transportation and distribution of Qi, blood and body fluid may ensue to result in diseases. Therefore, the disharmony between viscera, and disturbances of Qi, blood and body fluid can be corrected by regulating the channels and collaterals.

The mechanism of massotherapy in the treatment of diabetes is that the pressing, rubbing, pushing, grasping, and pressure-rubbing manipulations which act directly on the acupoints and muscles along the Twelve Regular Channels produce mechanic stimulations to remove the obstruction in the channels and collaterals, promote the flow of Qi and blood in them and to produce therapeutic effects. The dredging of the channels and collaterals enables the transportation and distribution of body fluid to return to normal, so that the heat will be removed and body fluids normalised to relieve the symptoms of thirst due to insufficiency of body fluids, and dryness-heat. In a protracted case of diabetes, because of the unsmooth flow of Qi and blood and blood stasis in the Yin collaterals, complications of microangiopathy and neuropathy may occur, marked by numbness and pain in the extremities. Massotherapy is effective in preventing and curing complications of microangiopathy and neuropathy because it renders the channels and collaterals clear by dredging them, smoothing circulation of Qi and blood and promoting blood circulation to eliminate blood stasis. Besides insufficiency of body fluid, excess of heat and unsmooth circulation of Qi and blood, the imbalance between Yin and Yang is another important pathogenic factor. By massage with the hands on the corresponding acupoints and channels and collaterals, massotherapy can guide Yin to join in Yang, and vice versa, and thus lead to the balance between Yin and Yang. Also through the stimulation by various massage manipulations on a local area of the body, the channels and collaterals are excited by the stimulant signals from the body surface to change the condition of the whole body, restoring the normal transportation and distribution of Yin, Yang, Qi, blood, and body fluid, and the coordinating relationships between the viscera, channels and collaterals, and Yin and Yang so that the excessive heat can be eliminated, the body fluid normalized and the symptoms of diabetes improved.

It is proved by modern medical research that massotherapy cures diabetes through comprehensive actions. It has been proved by the preliminary research that massage can improve the symptoms of diabetes, lower the glucose content in blood and urine and has some effects in the prevention and treatment of diabetic complications of microangiopathy and neuropathy, and therefore, as an adjuvant therapy, massage is recommended in the prevention and treatment of diabetes.

Clinical Application of Massotherapy

1. The indications and contraindications of massotherapy

(1) It is suitable for non-insulin-dependent diabetics, especially the levis-moderate and obese types.

(2) It is suitable for diabetics with complications of microangiopathy and neuropathy marked by numbness and pain in the limbs.

(3) It can also be used, along with insulin therapy, in the treatment of insulin-dependent diabetics whose condition is stable with little changes in blood glucose concentration.

(4) It should be used scrupulously in the treatment of severe diabetes or diabetes with unstable blood glucose level.

(5) It should never be used when a diabetic patient has developed severe cardiac, cerebral or renal complications, diabetic acidosis and skin infections. As for a diabetic during pregnancy, massotherapy should be prescribed very cautiously or forbidden. Massage on the abdomen in particular is forbidden.

2. Strength, duration and common lubricants of massage

(1) Strength of massage: Since most diabetics are poor in health, the massotherapy should be carried out in an orderly way and step by step in terms of manipulations. At the beginning, mild manipulations should be used, and then enforced gradually. Manipulations with great force should not be applied until the patient's constitution has been improved. A treatment should begin with mild manipulations and intensified gradually. Before completion of a treatment, the strength of manipulations should be reduced slowly from the strongest to mildest and cease in the end. The pressing and rubbing manipulations on an acupoint should be stopped when the patient has got the sensation of "arrival of Qi", that is, a soreness and distention sensetion or sometimes a radiating soreness and numbness sensation. If there is only

pain without such soreness-distention sensation, it is indicated that either the strength of the manipulation is too great or the location of acupoint is not accurate. Vibrating and kneading manipulations can also be incorporated into the pressing and rubbing manipulations so as to prolong or slow the process of "arrival of Qi".

(2) Duration of massage: In general, single-location massage takes about 15 minutes, and multiple-location massage, about 30 minutes. A course of massotherapy usually consists of no more than 15 times. If the course is too long, the curative effects will only be lessened rather than enhanced. There should be an interval of 3-5 days between two courses. Moreover, the time needed for massotherapy should be flexibly decided on the basis of the degree of urgency of the patient's condition and the severity of symptoms. As a rule, the time for each treatment is 15-30 minutes, once every day or every other day. 7-12 times constitute a course and another 1-2 courses are given after the first course depending on the condition of diseases. When necessary, even more courses can be given.

(3) The common lubricants for massage: When the pushing, rubbing and kneading manipulations are employed in clinics, in order to reduce the resistance from friction, heighten the curative effect and protect skin, the massagist often needs to put some lubricant on his hand and the area to be manipulated. Clinically, the common lubricants used are:

① Talc powder or toilet powder: They have certain water-absorbent, cooling and skin-lubricating effects.

② Mentha water: A small amount of peppermint is soaked in boiling water and when the water gets cold, strain the soak free from peppermint for use. It is suitable to be used in summer for its cooling and antipyretic effects.

③ Sesame oil: It has the effects of removing heat and wind, regulating blood, relieving pain and correcting deficiency.

④ Conducting oil: Being a compound oil blended up with wintergreen oil, glycerin, turpentine oil, alcohol, and distilled water, it is marked by good repercussive and analgesic effects and is good for diabetics with angioneurotic complications.

3. The common massage methods in the treatment of diabetes

(1) Self-massage: It refers to the massage in which a diabetic himself stimulates the specific locations on the body surface with proper massage manipulations. This method is easy to be adhered to for the virtues of freedom from time limitation and inconvenience of having to go to hospital.

Prescription 1: Press and knead Feishu and Weishu; knead and scrub Shenshu; rub Zhongwan; knead Qihai; press and knead Shousanli; grasp Hegu; grasp and press Neiguan and Waiguan; press and knead Zusanli; knead and press Sanyinjiao. The massage should be done in the above order, 20-30 times each point, both in the morning and evening, 30 minutes each time.

In case of diabetes mainly involving the upper Jiao marked by polydipsia and excessive thirst, on the basis of the above prescription, press Dazhui with a finger, and grasp and press Chize. In case of diabetes mainly involving the middle Jiao marked by polyphagia and bulimia, press Taichong with a finger, and nip and knead Neiting. For diabetes involving the lower Jiao characterized by polyuria and soreness in the waist, scrub Dazhui, press and knead Mingmen, grasp and press Taixi and Kunlun, and scrub Yongquan.

Massage on Feishu, Yishu, Pishu, Shenshu, Hegu, Quchi, Zusanli, and Sanyinjiao is also beneficial for the disease. These points should be kneaded and pressed with the palmar side of the thumb first with mild strength, and gradually from mild to great strength, from the trunk to the limbs and to the extent of soreness and distention sensation. Each point should be massaged for one minute.

Prescription 2: Grasp the limbs. Sit upright and put the hand on the thigh with the thumb on one side and the other four fingers on the other side, grasp and nip the legs gently from upper parts to the lower parts, i.e. from the groin to the ankle. Grasp and nip the anterior side of the legs for 5-10 times and then the posterior side for the same number. Then grasp and nip the left arm with the right hand from the shoulder to the wrist for 10-20 times. Massage the right arm with the left hand in the same way. This massage can be done 2-3 times a day.

Prescription 3: Knead acupoint Lianquan. Sit upright with the face slightly upward. Put the palmar side of the thumb on Lianquan and that of the forefinger on Chengjiang to knead and press them clockwise first with mild strength, which is gradually increased to be great. The massage should be continued till there is a local soreness and distention sensation. The massage can be done 2-3 times a day.

(2) Massage by the doctor: Also known as passive massage, it refers to the massage manipulations performed on diabetics by doctors according to massage theories. This is the principal form of massotherapy. Passive massage is mainly used to treat diabetes but can also be used for health preservation of diabetics.

Prescription 1: It consists mainly of massage on the channel points. The points often used are Geshu, Yishu, Ganshu, Danshu, Pishu, Weishu, Shenshu, etc. The basic manipulations are pushing with one-finger meditation, nipping, kneading, twisting, rubbing and pulling. The massage operation is as follows:

① The patient lies on the back and the doctor presses and rubs the patient's abdomen for about 5 minutes.

② Then the patient lies on the stomach. The doctor pushes, with one-finger meditation manipulation, the Urinary Bladder Channel on the two sides, to and fro between Geshu and Shenshu with the local pressure pain point or points as the focus of treatment. The treatment lasts about 10 minutes, followed by scrubbing the Urinary Bladder Channel till the operated part gets warm.

③ Nip and knead the intersecting area of the palm center and the middle crease of the fourth metacarpal for 5 minutes. This is the pancreatic reflecting area on the hand. While nipping and kneading, the doctor should concentrate on the patient's upper abdomen, imagining that his treatment is producing effect. In this way, the patient may have a warm and comfortable feeling there.

④ Nip and knead the medial margin of the sole at the first metatarsal capitulum for 5 minutes because it is the pancreatic reflecting region on the foot. While nipping and kneading, the doctor's mind should also concentrate on the patient's upper abdomen to produce a soreness-distention sensation there, which will disappear after treatment.

Prescription 2: The choice of points depends on the differentiation of the syndromes. For diabetes involving the upper Jiao, Feishu, Taiyuan, Yishu and Lianquan are of choice; for diabetes involving the middle Jiao, Weishu, Pishu, Yishu, Neiting and Sanyinjiao, and for diabetes involving the lower Jiao, Shenshu, Taixi, Yishu, Rangu and Xingjian may be selected. In case of excessive thirst and dry throat, Jinjin and Yuye are to be added. In case of bulimia and polyphagia, also massage Zhongwan and Zusanli. In the presence of dizziness and blurred vision, also massage Taiyang and Guangming, and in the presence of insufficiency of Yang and cold in the stomach, massage Mingmen and Guanyuan as well. Different manipulation methods should be used for different points. The massage should begin with knocking and twisting manipulations, and then use kneading and vibrating and finally complete by pushing with one-finger meditation. As a rule, gentle manipulations are first used followed by powerful ones. The massage session lasts 10-20 minutes and one session is given both in the morning and evening.

Prescription 3: The massage on the abdomen is the principal treatment to be supplemented by massage on other parts, channels, collaterals and points. The treatment is done in the following manner:

① Massage on the abdomen: The patient lies on the back with the hands lying straight on either side of the body and relaxed. The doctor stands on the patient's right to operate. First, knead and press Lanmen, Jianli, Qihai, Daimai, Zhangmen, Liangmen and Tianshu in clockwise movements, and grasp and lift the Ren

Channel. The treatment should be done mainly with uniform reinforcing-reducing manipulations for 15-20 minutes and the points should be pressed and rubbed in the order. Then apply special treatment. For example, if excessive thirst and polydipsia are present, knead and press left Liangmen and left Zhangmen area repeatedly with reduction manipulation for 3-5 minutes; in the presence of polyphagia and polydipsia, the points Zhongwan and Jianli should be kneaded and pressed repeatedly for 2-3 minutes with reduction manipulation or combined manipulations of regulation and reinforcement; in case of polyuria, the massage should be made mainly on the areas round Shuifen, Guanyuan and Zhongji by kneading and pressing repeatedly with reinforcement manipulation for 3-5 minutes.

② Pushing and pressing the back and waist: The patient takes sitting or prone position and the massagist stands at a proper position behind the patient, and massages from the upper to the lower parts. Push and press Jianjing, Yamen, Fengfu, Dazhui, Fengmen, Feishu, Gaohuang, Pishu and Shenshu in the above order for 3-5 minutes, mainly with flat pushing and two-direction pushing; then press the points on the back. Press Feishu, Xinshu, Geshu, Ganshu and Pishu to treat diabetes involving the upper Jiao; press Weishu, Pishu, Ganshu and Shenshu to treat diabetes involving the middle Jiao, and Shenshu, Feishu and Ganshu for diabetes involving the lower Jiao. Push and press repeatedly plus grasping and kneading for 5-10 minutes.

③ Local massage: As far as diabetes involving the upper Jiao is concerned, in addition to pushing and pressing the Feishu region, Zusanli should also be pushed and foulaged, and Yanglingquan should be plucked with reducing manipulation. For diabetes involving the middle Jiao, the center of the sole should also be rubbed, Sanyinjiao and Taixi should be massaged with digital press. For diabetes involving the lower Jiao, the waist should also be rubbed, the buttocks should be grasped, Feishu and Gaohuang, digital-pressed, and Jianjing and the shoulders kneaded.

(3) Massage of digital acupoint pressure with Qigong: As a

combination of Qigong and massage, it has a desirable effect on levis-moderate diabetes. The operation is performed in three steps:

① Starting posture: Stand quiet and relaxed, breathe out slowly 3 times, and open and close the middle Dantian 3 times.

② Massage with Qigong: Press and rub Chengjiang, Zhongwan, Guanyuan, Qimen and Shenshu in the listed order.

③ Ending posture: Open and close the middle Dantian 3 times and breathe out slowly 3 times. The three steps should be repeated 3 times on end. Before ending the practice, dry-wash the face. A session of the practice should be done both in the early morning and evening, about 1 hour each time. Half an hour's Qigong training for regulating breath and replenishing Qi is preferred before acupoint massage for 2-3 times.

Points of Attention in the Treatment of Diabetes with Massotherapy.

1. Massotherapy is a method in which various operations are performed chiefly by hand manipulations. The skills of manipulation, therefore, bear direct influence on the therapeutic effects. Whether the massage manipulations are right or improper is often one of the key factors that will lead to success or failure in the treatment of a disease. Therefore, the massage manipulations must be accurate, consistent, powerful and gentle, and should be performed with concentration of mind, concurrent flow of Qi and adequate strength.

2. Generally after a massage treatment, the patient feels comfortable and relaxed, However, there are patients who have discomfort such as soreness and pain at the manipulated regions. This is a normal reaction which will be improved on the second treatment and disappear on the third time of treatment. The patient will then feel comfortable and relaxed.

3. In order to prevent any discomfort, it is advisable for the patient not to be treated with massotherapy within 1 hour before

and after meal. After a treatment, the patient should have a little rest or some movements before leaving the clinic.

4. During massage treatment, the lubricants should be ready and the massagist should have his nails well trimmed. Neither should he wear his watch so that any injury to the patient's skin which might interfer with the treatment can be avoided.

5. Massotherapy has certain curative effects on mild and moderate types of diabetes and can also be used as an adjuvant treatment for severe diabetes. It must, however, go along with other therapies such as dietotherapy and pharmacotherapy. Otherwise, it is very difficult to achieve good therapeutic effects.

Editor-in-Chief: Cheng Yichun
Deputy Editor-in-Chief: Qian Qiuhai Yin Yihui
　Zhang Dengbu Feng Jianhua
Authors: Cheng Yichun Feng Jianhua Li Huadong
　Qian Qiuhai Wang Guocai Xu Yunsheng Yin Yihui
　Zhang Dengbu

糖尿病非药物疗法

程益春　主编
张玉玺
路玉滨　译

责任编辑　王为珍
　　　　　仲彭军

*

山东科学技术出版社出版
中国济南玉函路16号　邮政编码250002
山东新华印刷厂印刷
中国国际图书贸易总公司发行
中国北京车公庄西路35号
北京邮政信箱第399号　邮政编码100044

*

1997年6月(大32开)1版1次
ISBN 7-5331-1894-4
R·551
03000
14-E-3036P